The Easy
ANTI-INFLAMMATORY COOKBOOK

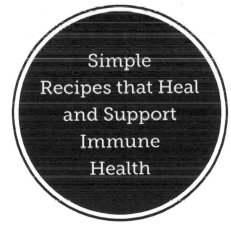

Simple Recipes that Heal and Support Immune Health

MOLLY THOMPSON

NEW SHOE PRESS

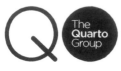

Brimming with creative inspiration, how-to projects, and useful information to enrich your everyday life, quarto.com is a favorite destination for those pursuing their interests and passions.

First Published in 2023 by New Shoe Press, an imprint of The Quarto Group, 100 Cummings Center, Suite 265-D, Beverly, MA 01915, USA.
T (978) 282-9590 F (978) 283-2742 Quarto.com

New Shoe Press titles are also available at discount for retail, wholesale, promotional, and bulk purchase. For details, contact the Special Sales Manager by email at specialsales@quarto.com or by mail at The Quarto Group, Attn: Special Sales Manager, 100 Cummings Center, Suite 265-D, Beverly, MA 01915, USA.

ISBN: 978-0-7603-7969-1
eISBN: 978-0-7603-7970-7

Library of Congress Cataloging-in-Publication Data available.

The content in this book was previously published in *The Anti-Inflammatory Diet Made Simple* (Fair Winds Press 2021) by Molly Thompson.

Cover Image: Molly Thompson
Photography: Molly Thompson

The information in this book is for educational purposes only. It is not intended to replace the advice of a physician or medical practitioner. Please see your health-care provider before beginning any new health program.

To Zach and Cooper,

You inspire me in the kitchen and bring joy to every part of my life. Cooking with you and sharing meals around the table are my favorite memories of all.

Contents

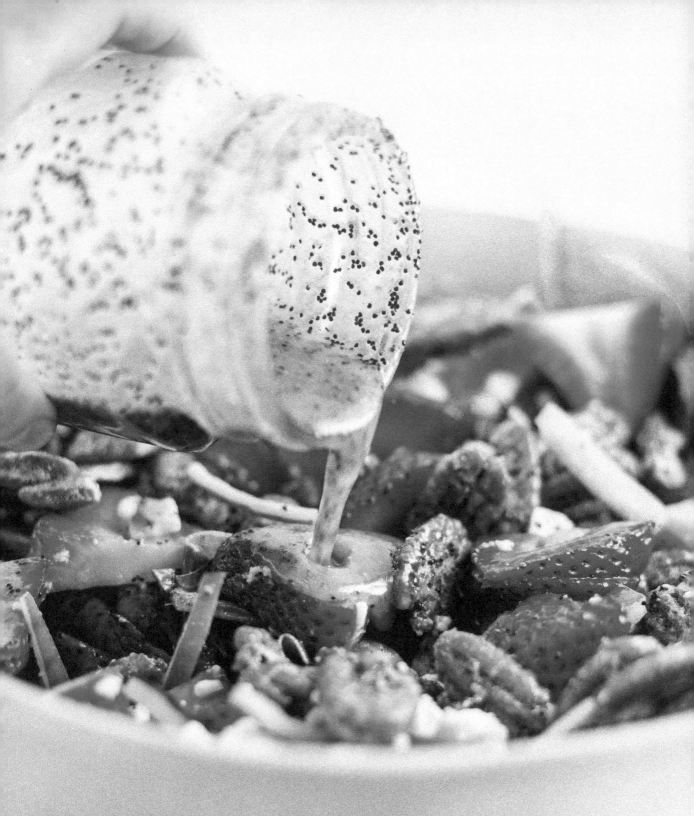

Strawberry–Spinach Salad, page 126

Introduction

I remember getting my first cookbook on my thirteenth birthday from my best friend. I opened it up and dove right in, flipping through the pages and whipping up my favorite recipes. The banana bread and blueberry scones were especially good.

I remember my mom asking me to make them again so she could take them to work and share with her friends. From that moment on, I was hooked. Hooked on creating something out of nothing but simple ingredients. It's amazing how five ingredients put together can become a meal that nourishes your entire family. I loved that feeling of accomplishment when a dish was done and seeing people's joy when they ate the food I had put all my love into.

I started my blog, What Molly Made, to share that passion with the world. Beyond that, I wanted to share recipes that make busy lives easier and help people bring their families together over a common love language: food!

When I was diagnosed with polycystic ovarian syndrome (PCOS) in the summer of 2018, my blog and recipes were about to take an unexpected turn. I was feeling overwhelmed, upset, angry, and confused by symptoms that made me feel like I wasn't myself. I wasn't sure where to go for advice besides turning to a Google search with panic. I went from website to website and doctor to doctor, all the while thinking there had to be a better way than medication to heal. Eventually, I found myself at the office of a functional medicine certified nurse practitioner, whose role is to help find the root cause of a medical issue or disease rather than treating the symptoms. So, instead of treating the symptoms of my PCOS with medication, I would instead find the root cause of my PCOS and reverse it with lifestyle changes.

Throughout a growing relationship with my functional certified nurse practitioner, I was introduced to the anti-inflammatory diet, which was presented to me as a way of eating to heal your body from the inside out. I knew that eating well was important to overall health, but I didn't understand the power that diet can have to heal stubborn symptoms (not just PCOS, but headaches, joint pain, and more!).

So, wait, you're telling me I can reverse my symptoms and feel good again all while eating great-tasting food? Sign me up!

Soon after I focused on incorporating anti-inflammatory foods into my life, I noticed a huge improvement. My symptoms were being reversed and I started to feel like myself again. If you know anything about PCOS, you know it can be a major factor in infertility. I'm happy to say that I'm sitting here writing this chapter with my four-month-old sleeping in my arms. All of this happened not because of medicine, but because of food.

To me, it's not a "diet" in the sense that our culture uses the word. It's just a way of eating that helps me feel healthy. I became empowered to change a diagnosis some doctors told me could never go away.

I'm a firm believer in using your pain and struggles to help those who are going through similar challenges. And my faith has taught me that I could use my story to make a difference. I started creating anti-inflammatory recipes on What Molly Made. I started talking about PCOS, and I found a community of people who understand it, who know the hurt, who long for a better answer, and who have faith in themselves to overcome the challenges. It's not just my passion to cook, but my purpose to share recipes that are not only easy and exciting but also make people feel good from the inside out.

My hope is that the recipes in this book bless your home and your bodies. Whatever season you're walking through, whether it's a difficult diagnosis or a journey to feel better, I want this book to be a tool to help you feel your best and nourish your body with recipes you look forward to making. These recipes do so much more than fill your stomach with yummy food—although they sure do that, too! They have the power to heal and the power to bring people together.

Anti-Inflammatory Recipes Key

Use the following symbols to see how each recipe adheres to the anti-inflammatory diet, with markers such as refined sugar-free, and incorporates other eating habits and allergies, such as vegan and gluten-free, as well.

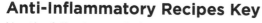

DF	GF	LC	P	SF	VG	V
Dairy-free	Gluten-free	Low carb	Paleo	Refined sugar-free	Vegan	Vegetarian

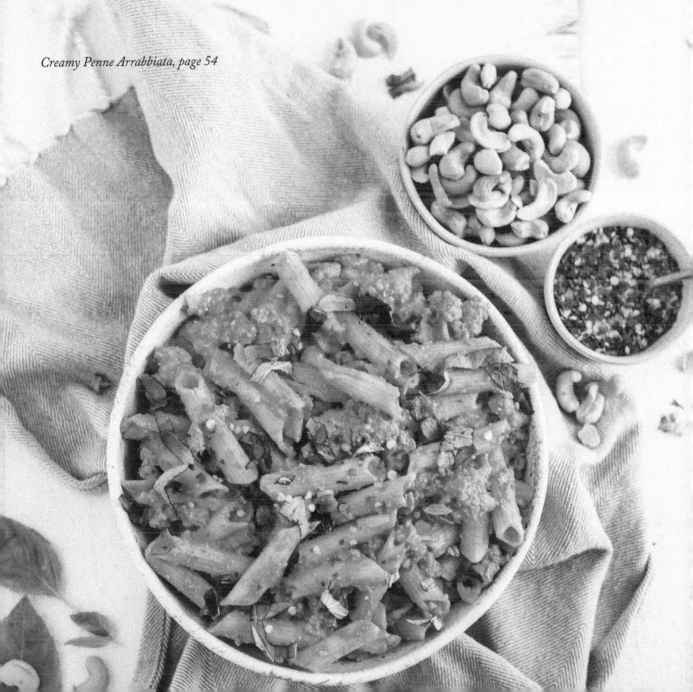

The Basics of the Anti-Inflammatory Diet

Creamy Penne Arrabbiata, page 54

Understanding Inflammation

What Is Chronic Inflammation?

You've probably heard the term *inflammation* before, but you may not understand how inflammation is related to food and the way you feel from day to day.

When you think of inflammation, maybe you think of the pain and redness that occurs on your skin because of a rash or an allergic reaction. If you've ever broken a bone, been stung by a bee, or cut your finger, you may be familiar with your body's immune response to protect itself. The inflammation that occurs is an essential survival mode that helps our bodies fight off harmful microbes and begin to repair itself. This acute inflammation is great at protecting our bodies in those instances. But too much of a good thing can be harmful, and that's where chronic inflammation comes in.

Our bodies can have an inflammatory response to the food we eat and, over time, maintain a prolonged inflammatory state, which can have adverse effects on our health. But, as we shall see, food has the power not only to cause inflammation but also to fight inflammation.

What Are the Symptoms of Chronic Inflammation?

Here are some telltale signs of inflammation to mention at your next healthcare appointment:

- Digestive issues (leaky gut, bloating, gas, irritable bowel syndrome [IBS], constipation)
- Headaches
- Hormone imbalances (irregular cycles, polycystic ovarian syndrome [PCOS])
- Autoimmune diseases (Hashimoto's disease, rheumatoid arthritis)
- Skin issues (acne, psoriasis, eczema)
- Mood disorders (anxiety, depression)
- Trouble sleeping
- Trouble losing weight

If you are suffering from one or more of these issues (in the absence of symptoms pointing to another medical issue), you can request blood work from your healthcare provider to test for the presence of inflammation in your body. Your CRP (C-reactive protein) and GGT (gamma-glutamyl transferase) numbers are markers for inflammation.

Why Is Reducing Inflammation Important?

Reducing chronic inflammation in your body is important because it's not meant to be there! In the presence of inflammation, your body cannot function to its full potential. By reducing inflammation, you can ease inflammatory-caused issues like those listed previously.

Above all, when you're free of inflammation, you feel your best. When you feel your best, you live with purpose, and your cup is overflowing to help others. And that just creates a ripple effect.

Foods That Help Reduce Inflammation

The key to adapting to this new way of eating is to think in terms of adding beneficial foods to your diet, rather than restricting it. When you choose foods that make you feel good, the inflammatory foods are simply no longer in the picture.

Here are some of the foods that are especially helpful for fighting inflammation:

Vegetables: Veggies provide important nutrients, such as vitamin C, folate, and magnesium. They feed your beneficial gut bacteria and contain phytonutrients (plant chemicals) that fight inflammation. In order to get as wide a variety of nutrients as possible, try to eat a rainbow of vegetables, like carrots, spinach, bell peppers, and butternut squash.

Fruits: Fiber- and antioxidant-rich fruits are great for inflammation. As with veggies, choose a variety of colors of fruits, like apples, blueberries, pomegranates, and bananas.

Whole grains: Focus on eating gluten-free whole grains, like quinoa, rice, amaranth, and oats. (Oats are naturally gluten-free, but be sure to check that the label says "certified gluten-free," since cross-contamination can occur during processing.)

Healthy fats: Omega-3 fatty acids help fight inflammation. These fats can be found in abundance in salmon and other seafood, as well as in certain plant-based foods, like avocado, coconut oil, and chia seeds.

Spices: Spices are not only good for fighting inflammation but they also make food taste better! Two great anti-inflammatory spices to try are turmeric and cinnamon. And although they're not technically spices, ginger and garlic are often used in recipes to add flavor, and both also have strong anti-inflammatory properties.

Fermented foods: My favorite fermented foods are kombucha, sauerkraut, and apple cider vinegar. They're naturally full of probiotics that can help heal the gut.

Bone broth: On top of fighting inflammation, bone broth is great for your gut and boosts immunity. It's also rich in amino acids and minerals. You can cook noodles and rice with bone broth or swap in bone broth for regular chicken broth in any recipe.

Beans and legumes: In addition to being anti-inflammatory, beans are full of fiber, protein, and magnesium. If you're new to beans, start by trying lentils, chickpeas, or black beans.

Foods That Can Contribute to Inflammation

Just as certain foods can fight inflammation, other foods can contribute to it. Not everyone has the same response to every food, but it helps to know which foods are common triggers for inflammation.

Here are some of the foods that can contribute to inflammation:

Gluten: Gluten, found in wheat and some other grains, is one of the most common food sensitivities. It affects people differently, but research has found that gluten has an inflammatory response in six out of ten women.

Dairy: The inflammatory part of dairy is a protein called A1 casein; it stimulates the immune system to create those inflammatory messengers. Dairy is the second most common food sensitivity.

Very Berry Ginger Smoothie, page 135

Sugar: Sugar, in its many forms, can cause tissue damage and insulin resistance because it generates inflammation in the liver. And in women, too much insulin can impair ovulation.

Alcohol: Alcohol shrinks the hippocampus, impairs the healthy clearance of estrogen, causes insulin resistance, damages gut bacteria, prevents nutrient absorption, impairs detoxification, and depletes an anti-inflammatory molecule called glutathione. In addition, it is often consumed by mixing with sugary beverages, compounding the effects.

Vegetable oils: Many vegetable oils, such as canola oil and corn oil, contain omega-6 fatty acids, which can promote inflammation when used in large amounts. Great oils to cook with instead include olive oil, avocado oil, and coconut oil.

It's Not Always Black and White

It's tempting to read all this information and start creating "bad food" and "good food" lists in your head. If you're anything like me, maybe you've struggled with restrictive diets all your life and find that foods that are off-limits trigger a negative response emotionally. Or maybe you're at a restaurant and there's a killer cheese board calling your name.

If that's the case, take a bite! Don't ever be afraid to enjoy life through food and experiences. But it's also important to be mindful of what makes you feel your best. I noticed a massive shift when I started to think about the food I eat in terms of my long-term health and how it makes me feel rather than how it makes me look.

I followed a pretty strict anti-inflammatory protocol for thirty days, in addition to doing a food sensitivity test. After that, I slowly reintroduced foods back into my diet to see which ones made me feel inflamed. By just being mindful, I now know which foods cause gastrointestinal disturbances or make me feel "blah" and which ones make me feel my best. As with many things, find what works for you!

The recipes in this book focus on incorporating all the best inflammation-fighting foods and provide tasty, easy-to-find alternatives to foods that may contribute to inflammation in your body.

WHAT IS PALEO?

The paleo diet is similar to an anti-inflammatory way of eating where gluten, dairy, and refined sugars are avoided with a focus on whole, clean foods. They're almost used synonymously, but anti-inflammatory meals include grains like rice and gluten-free oats.

Key Ingredients and Cooking Essentials

I love to cook, and over the years I've found that there are some kitchen tools I can't live without. Whether it's a simple breakfast for one or an elaborate dinner for friends, these are the tools I use regularly.

Cooking Essentials

Here are some of my favorite kitchen tools:

Sharp knives: I use a large chef's knife and a paring knife daily. You'll need them to cut and chop all the fruits and vegetables in this book!

Stand mixer or handheld mixer: Either type of mixer can be used for most recipes, but I prefer to use my stand mixer for large-batch desserts or when I need my hands free.

Cast-iron or ceramic skillet: A well-seasoned cast-iron or ceramic skillet is the best choice for recipes that need to go from stovetop to oven and back. Many other skillets are also oven-safe; check the manufacturer's recommendations if you're not sure.

Rimmed baking sheets: Also called sheet pans, these are indispensable for roasting veggies and baking cookies. I highly recommend having at least two of these on hand.

Blender (preferably high-speed) or food processor: These appliances make quick work of sauces, soups, salsas, and more.

Nut milk bag or cheesecloth: If you find you're making nut milk frequently, I recommend buying a nut milk bag; otherwise, a few layers of cheesecloth will work just as well. Either will allow you to strain small objects from a liquid.

Slow cooker: What could be better than throwing all your ingredients into a slow cooker and coming home to a finished meal?

Pressure cooker: The new breed of multicookers allow you to make an entire meal with the sauté mode and pressure cook settings. Most models also have a slow cooker option!

Key Ingredients

The anti-inflammatory diet is made up of real, whole foods. Ones you can find growing in the earth and around the periphery of the grocery store. If a product's ingredient list contains only one thing, or better yet, if it doesn't have an ingredient list, it's probably a great ingredient for this diet.

However, some ingredients in the recipes that follow may be new to you. They are available at Whole Foods Market and many well-stocked grocery stores, and you can find them all online. Here are some of my favorite ingredients to keep on hand for preparing anti-inflammatory meals:

Gluten-free pasta: My favorite pastas are made from brown rice and chickpeas. You can find both options at any well-stocked grocery store. Just be sure to check the package directions, as cooking instructions may vary.

Fats: My favorite fats to cook with are coconut oil, avocado oil, and olive oil. Coconut oil is my choice for making baked goods because it's solid at room temperature. I use avocado oil when I'm cooking at a high temperature. I reserve extra-virgin olive oil to make salad dressings.

Full-fat coconut milk: Canned coconut milk comes with a thick layer of coconut cream on the top. The recipe will specify whether you are supposed to use just the cream from the top or shake the can first to mix it with the milk. This is a great dairy-free option to thicken creamy soups, sauces, and dips.

Paleo mayo: Mayonnaise made with pasteurized eggs and avocado oil is a great alternative to the traditional kind made with vegetable oil and sugar. My favorite brand is Primal Kitchen. Most traditional mayos will have canola oil and some sort of sweetener—usually refined sugar—so choosing a paleo mayo means it's made with a clean oil like avocado oil and no sweetener.

Coconut aminos: This product is a great substitute for soy sauce that's gluten- and soy-free. A popular brand is Bragg.

Chocolate chips: Grab a dairy-free brand like Enjoy Life or Lily's chocolate made with stevia and you'll be ready to whip up some Double Chocolate Banana Blender Muffins (page 24) for a snack or dessert.

Nutritional yeast: This unique ingredient is a deactivated yeast, typically sold in the form of flakes in the bulk section. With its nutty flavor, it makes a great substitute for grated cheese in dishes like Spicy Black Bean Nachos (page 123) and Roasted Summer Vegetable Pesto Pasta (page 43). Nutritional yeast is a complete protein and also contains B vitamins and trace minerals like zinc and magnesium.

Chicken and vegetable broths: I always keep at least a couple of cartons of broth on hand for quick soups and sauces. If you can find bone broth, even better! It helps heal the gut.

Protein: Try to purchase high-quality meat and seafood whenever possible. A great option is to sign up for a high-quality meat delivery service or enroll in a CSA (community supported agriculture) program with a local farm. Organic, free-range chicken, grass-fed beef and pork, and wild-caught seafood are optimal protein options for an anti-inflammatory diet.

Miscellaneous pantry items: Spices, nuts and seeds, nut butters, rice, quinoa, canned beans, and canned tomatoes are great to have on hand.

Flours and Starches

To make recipes that are gluten-free, you'll want to stock your pantry with a variety of alternative flour products:

Cassava flour: Cassava flour is gaining momentum as a gluten-free, grain-free, nut-free flour alternative since it is the most similar in structure to wheat flour. It comes from the cassava root, which is peeled, dried, and ground. You'll use cassava flour to make my Sweet Potato Gnocchi (page 44).

Tapioca flour/starch: Tapioca flour also comes from the cassava root, but instead of the whole root, the starch is extracted from the root through washing and pulping. It's a great alternative to cornstarch for thickening soups, like the Tuscan Sausage and Cauliflower Soup (page 76), or it can be mixed with other flours for baked goods.

Coconut flour: Coconut flour is ground from dried coconut meat and thus has a slight coconut flavor. It is often combined with other flours for baking. Beware of using coconut flour in a recipe that doesn't call for it! Coconut flour absorbs a lot of moisture and can leave your baked goods dry if you don't have the right ratio of dry ingredients and liquids.

Almond flour: Also known as almond meal, this popular flour alternative is made from blanched (skinless) almonds. It has a fine texture and light color, and its more neutral flavor pairs well with other flours, especially coconut flour.

Arrowroot flour/starch: Much like tapioca flour, arrowroot is a powder derived from a plant—in this case, a tropical tuber. It can be substituted for cornstarch to thicken sauces and soups or combined with other flours to make baked goods.

Sweeteners

Just because you'll be avoiding refined sugar in the anti-inflammatory diet doesn't mean you can't add sweetness to your life! Of course, being mindful of the amount of sweetener you use is important, but a delicious baked good should be something everyone can enjoy. There are several options:

Maple syrup: Be sure to buy pure maple syrup—and get an extra-large jug because it goes so well in sweet and savory recipes, like Paleo Coffee Cake Doughnuts with Crumble Topping (page 23) or BBQ Chicken Zucchini Boats (page 68).

Honey: Be sure to get raw honey or manuka honey, which is said to have antibacterial properties. It's a great way to sweeten up your nighttime Golden Turmeric-Honey Latte (page 140).

Coconut sugar: This sugar is made from coconut palm sap and can be used to sweeten a recipe without the runny texture from syrup or honey.

CHAPTER TWO

Breakfast

Sweet Potato Waffle Breakfast Sandwich, page 30

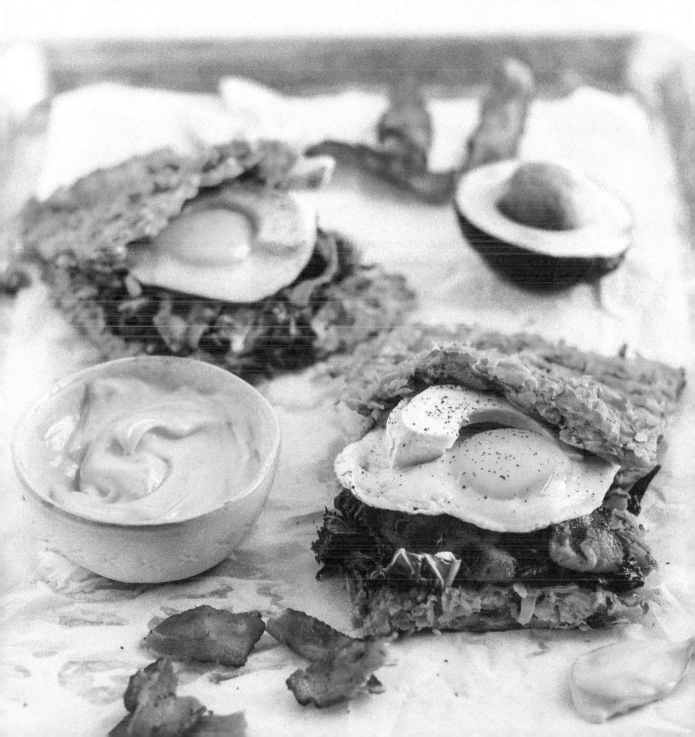

Banana Oatmeal Pancakes

These pancakes are a gluten-free, dairy-free take on the classic weekend staple. A slow Saturday morning calls for a stack of these easy pancakes. Throw everything in the blender and cook! You can even store them in the refrigerator for a simple weekday breakfast.

2¼ cups (180 g) gluten-free rolled oats

2 large ripe bananas

1 cup (237 ml) unsweetened vanilla nondairy milk

1 large egg

1 tablespoon (20 g) pure maple syrup or raw honey, plus more for serving (optional)

1 teaspoon pure vanilla extract

1½ teaspoons baking powder

½ teaspoon ground cinnamon

¼ teaspoon salt

1 teaspoon coconut oil, or more if needed

Sliced bananas, berries, nuts, and/or nut butter, for topping (optional)

—
Yield | 4 servings

Combine the oats, bananas, milk, egg, maple syrup, vanilla, baking powder, cinnamon, and salt in a blender and blend on high until the oats have broken down, 2 to 3 minutes.

Melt the coconut oil in a large skillet over medium-low heat. Working in batches, pour in ¼ cup (59 ml) of the batter for each pancake. Cook until the edges of the pancake are set and the top starts to bubble, 2 to 3 minutes, then flip and cook on the other side for another 2 to3 minutes. Repeat with the remaining batter, adding more oil if necessary.

Serve the pancakes hot with your favorite toppings.

PRO TIP!

If you like thicker pancakes, add an additional ¼ cup (20 g) oats to the blender. If you like them thinner, add an additional 2 to 3 tablespoons (30 to 45 ml) milk.

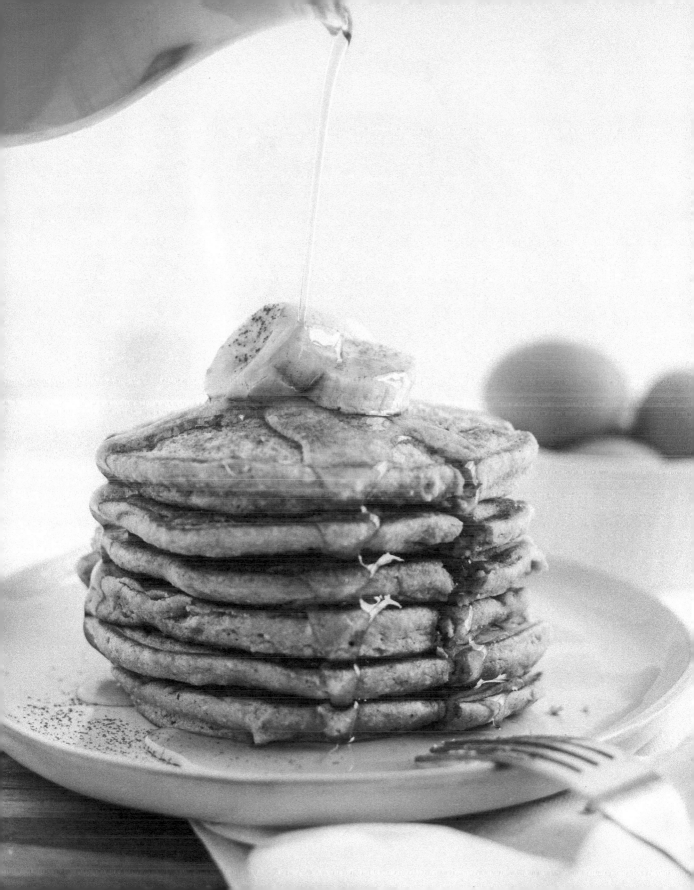

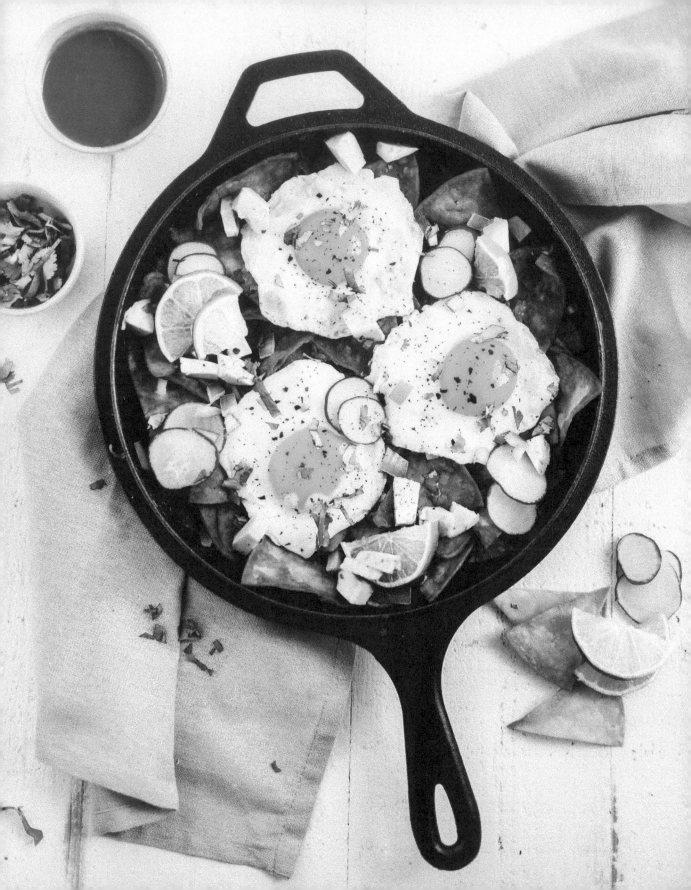

Chilaquiles Rojos with Eggs

In its most basic form, chilaquiles is a Mexican dish made with fried tortillas simmered in a red or green sauce. This dish is easy to make, affordable, and great for entertaining because it feeds a crowd.

8 corn tortillas

½ cup (118 ml) avocado oil or coconut oil

¼ teaspoon salt, plus more to taste

1 cup (237 ml) no-sugar-added red enchilada sauce

4 large eggs

¼ cup (40 g) dicedred onion

1 avocado, peeled, pitted, and chopped or sliced

2 radishes, thinly sliced

2 tablespoons (8 g) chopped fresh cilantro

1 lime, cut into 4 wedges

—

Yield | 4 servings

Preheat the oven to 425°F (220°C).

Stack the tortillas and cut them into 8 wedges. Heat the oil in a large cast-iron skillet over medium-high heat until it reaches 325°F (170°C) to 350°F (180°C). Working in batches, add the tortilla wedges, taking care not to crowd the pan. Cook until golden brown, 1 to 2 minutes, then flip and cook on the other side for another 1 to 2 minutes. Transfer the tortilla chips to paper towels and sprinkle with a pinch of salt.

Pour off the excess oil from the pan and add the enchilada sauce. Heat over medium-high heat for 2 to 3 minutes, then add the tortilla chips and toss to coat evenly and to slightly soften the chips. Crack the eggs on top and transfer the skillet to the oven. Bake for 7 to 8 minutes, until the eggs are set but still runny.

Serve topped with red onion, avocado, radish, and cilantro, with a squeeze of lime juice.

PRO TIP!

It's best to use an oil with a high smoke point for frying the tortillas. Avocado oil's smoke point is 520°F (270°C), and coconut oil's smoke point is 450°F (230°C).

Sweet Potato Toast 4 Ways

Are you a sweet or savory fan? These sweet potato toast recipes give you options for whatever mood you're in! And the "toast" is really as simple as popping a slice of sweet potato in the toaster. It's a gluten-free vehicle for all your favorite savory and sweet toppings. Each variation below makes enough to top 1 toast.

For the sweet potato toast:

1 large sweet potato

For the avocado and egg topping:

1 teaspoon coconut oil

1 large egg

½ avocado, peeled and pitted

Salt and black pepper, to taste

Chopped fresh parsley and/or crushed red pepper, for garnish

For the caramelized apple or banana topping:

2 teaspoons coconut oil

1 small apple, cored and thinly sliced, or 1 small banana, thinly sliced

2 teaspoons pure maple syrup

½ teaspoon ground cinnamon

1 tablespoon (15 g) cashew or almond butter

For the seedy avocado topping:

½ avocado, peeled and pitted

1 teaspoon pumpkin seeds

1 teaspoon sesame seeds

1 teaspoon sunflower seeds

½ teaspoon chia seeds

Salt and black pepper, to taste

Olive oil, for garnish

For the blueberry-almond topping:

2 tablespoons (30 g) almond butter

¼ cup (38 g) blueberries

½ teaspoon chia seeds

1 teaspoon raw honey

—

Yield | 4 sweet potato toasts

To make the toast, cut the sweet potato lengthwise into four ⅓-inch (8 mm) slices. Place the slices in the toaster and toast on high for 5 minutes. Check to see if they're fork-tender, and toast for a little longer if needed, taking care not to let them burn. (Alternatively, preheat the oven to 400°F [200°C] and bake the sweet potato slices on a parchment-lined rimmed baking sheet for 20 to 25 minutes.)

Avocado and Egg: Melt the coconut oil in a small skillet over medium-low heat. Add the egg and cook until the white is set, 3 to 5 minutes. Mash or slice the avocado, place it on the toasted sweet potato, and top with the fried egg. Season with salt and pepper, then garnish with parsley and crushed red pepper.

Caramelized Apple: Melt the coconut oil in a small skillet over medium heat. Add the apple or banana, maple syrup, and cinnamon and cook, stirring, until softened, 5 to 7 minutes. Spread the nut butter on the sweet potato toast and top with the caramelized apples.

Seedy Avocado: Slice or mash the avocado, place it on the sweet potato toast, and sprinkle with the seeds. Season with salt and pepper and drizzle olive oil on top.

Blueberry-Almond: Spread the almond butter on the sweet potato toast and top with the blueberries and chia seeds. Drizzle with the honey.

Blueberry Chia Jam

Skip the refined sugar and make your own healthy jam! The blueberries and chia seeds deliver powerful antioxidants and fiber. Dollop this jam on your favorite dairy-free yogurt or slather it on a paleo-friendly muffin.

2 cups (290 g) fresh blueberries

2 tablespoons (30 ml) water

1 tablespoon (20 g) raw honey or pure maple syrup, plus more to taste

2 tablespoons (16 g) chia seeds

1 tablespoon (15 ml) lemon juice

—

Yield | 1 cup (400 g)

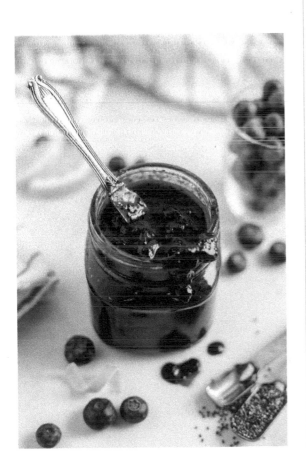

Combine the blueberries, water, and honey in a medium nonstick saucepan and heat over medium heat. Cook, stirring occasionally, until the blueberries turn darker and the liquid starts to bubble, about 5 minutes. As the blueberries begin to break down, use a wooden spoon or a silicone spatula to mash them, depending on how chunky you want your jam. Once bubbling, turn the heat down to low and continue to simmer and mash the blueberries for 5 more minutes, or until the mixture becomes thick.

Stir in the chia seeds and lemon juice. Taste and add more honey if you want it to be sweeter. Remove the pan from the heat and allow it to sit at room temperature for 10 to 15 minutes. Use immediately or store in an airtight container in the refrigerator for up to 10 days. As the jam cools it will get thicker.

ADD IT!

If blueberries aren't in season, you can make this jam with frozen blueberries. Just simmer the jam for an additional 5 minutes to reduce because frozen berries hold more moisture.

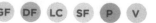
Roasted Cauliflower and Herb Quiche with Hash Brown Crust

A crispy, crunchy potato crust is a great anti-inflammatory alternative to the traditional pie crust in a quiche. An assortment of fresh herbs makes this healthy, protein-packed dish the star of any brunch menu—whether served warm or at cold.

For the roasted cauliflower:

3 cups (300 g) small cauliflower florets

2 tablespoons (30 ml) olive oil

1 teaspoon garlic powder

½ teaspoon salt

⅛ teaspoon black pepper

For the hash brown crust:

2 pounds (907 g) russet potatoes (4 medium), peeled and grated

1 teaspoon salt

¼ teaspoon black pepper

3 tablespoons (45 ml) olive oil

For the quiche:

8 large eggs

1 cup (237 ml) unsweetened nondairy milk

¼ cup (16 g) chopped fresh tarragon

2 tablespoons (8 g) minced fresh basil

2 tablespoons (8 g) minced fresh parsley

1 teaspoon salt

¼ teaspoon black pepper

Arugula, for topping

—
Yield | 8 servings

Preheat the oven to 350°F (180°C). Line a rimmed baking sheet with parchment paper or a silicone baking mat.

To make the roasted cauliflower, scatter the cauliflower florets on the prepared baking sheet, drizzle with the olive oil, and sprinkle with the garlic powder, salt, and pepper. Roast for 10 minutes, stir, and roast for about 10 more minutes, or until the cauliflower is fork-tender and browned around the edges.

To make the hash brown crust, place the grated potatoes on a large kitchen towel. Gather the edges of the towel around the potatoes and squeeze over the sink to extract as much liquid as possible. Transfer the potatoes to a bowl and season with the salt and pepper.

Heat the oil in a large oven-safe skillet over medium heat, swirling the pan so the oil coats the bottom and sides. Add the potatoes and press them down in a thin, even layer with the back of a spatula to form a crust on the bottom and sides of the skillet. Press and mold the potatoes for 10 to 12 minutes, until the edges are golden brown. Remove the pan from the heat.

To make the quiche, whisk together the eggs and milk in a large bowl. Add the tarragon, basil, parsley, salt and pepper, and whisk to combine. Add the roasted cauliflower, then pour the mixture on top of the crust.

Bake for 45 to 50 minutes, until the quiche is golden on the top and set in the center. Top with a handful of arugula and cut into wedges to serve.

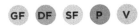

Paleo Coffee Cake Doughnuts with Crumble Topping

Here's a combination of everyone's two favorite breakfast treats: doughnuts and coffee cake! This heart-warming and sweet breakfast recipe pairs perfectly with a large cup of joe and a front porch with the sun rising. Store these in the freezer for a yummy doughnut any day of the week.

Nonstick cooking spray

For the crumble topping:

¾ cup (84 g) almond flour

3 tablespoons (24 g) tapioca flour

⅓ cup (67 g) coconut sugar

½ teaspoon ground cinnamon

¼ teaspoon salt

⅓ cup (75 g) coconut oil, at room temperature

For the doughnuts:

⅔ cup (82 g) coconut flour

¼ cup (32 g) tapioca flour

2 teaspoons ground cinnamon

½ teaspoon baking soda

¼ teaspoon salt

4 large eggs, at room temperature

½ cup (170 g) pure maple syrup

⅓ cup (77 ml) well-shaken canned full-fat coconut milk

2 tablespoons (28 g) coconut oil, melted and cooled slightly

1 teaspoon pure vanilla extract

For the maple icing (optional)

¼ cup (60 g) cashew or other nut butter, melted

2 tablespoons (16 g) tapioca flour

3 tablespoons (60 g) pure maple syrup

2 to 3 tablespoons (30 to 45 ml) water

—

Yield | 9 doughnuts

Preheat the oven to 350°F (180°C). Lightly grease 9 holes of a 12-mold doughnut pan with nonstick cooking spray.

To make the crumble topping, in a medium bowl, whisk together the almond flour, tapioca flour, coconut sugar, cinnamon, and salt. Add the solid coconut oil and use a pastry blender or two knives to cut it into the dry ingredients. Continue to blend until a crumbly mixture forms.

To make the doughnuts, in a medium bowl, whisk together the coconut flour, tapioca flour, cinnamon, baking soda, and salt.

Using a handheld mixer or a stand mixer fitted with the paddle attachment, beat together the eggs, maple syrup, coconut milk, coconut oil, and vanilla until fully combined and light yellow. Slowly beat the dry ingredients into the wet ingredients until completely incorporated, being careful not to overmix. Spoon the batter into 9 molds in the prepared doughnut pan, filling each to the top. Sprinkle the crumble topping on top of each. Bake for 22 to 25 minutes, until a toothpick inserted in the center comes out clean and the tops are a light golden brown. Cool the doughnuts in the pan for 15 minutes, then transfer to a wire rack to cool completely.

To make the maple icing, if desired, combine all the icing ingredients in a small bowl and mix well. Drizzle over the doughnuts.

> **PRO TIP!**
>
> If you make doughnuts often, you might want to invest in a silicone doughnut pan for easy removal.

Double Chocolate Banana Blender Muffins

With a special baking trick, these easy, flavor-packed muffins turn into sky-high bakery-style treats that really impress. Share with your friends or store them for an easy weekday breakfast.

Nonstick cooking spray

1½ cups (120 g) gluten-free rolled oats

⅓ cup (40 g) unsweetened cocoa powder

1 tablespoon (8 g) cornstarch

½ teaspoon baking soda

½ teaspoon salt

3 large overripe bananas

1 large egg

½ cup (118 ml) unsweetened nondairy milk

⅓ cup (115 g) raw honey or pure maple syrup

3 tablespoons (42 g) coconut oil, melted and cooled slightly

2 teaspoons pure vanilla extract

¾ cup (131 g) dairy-free chocolate chips

—

Yield | 12 muffins

Preheat the oven to 425°F (220°C). Line a standard muffin tin with cupcake liners and spray with nonstick cooking spray.

In a large bowl, whisk together the oats, cocoa powder, cornstarch, baking soda, and salt.

In a large blender, combine the bananas, egg, milk, honey, coconut oil, and vanilla. Blend on high until smooth and creamy, about 1 minute. Pour the wet ingredients into the dry ingredients and whisk until just combined, being careful not to overmix. Gently fold in the chocolate chips, saving a few for the top of each muffin.

Divide the batter evenly among the prepared muffin cups. Scatter a few of the reserved chocolate chips on top of each muffin.

Bake for 5 minutes, then reduce the heat to 350°F (180°C) and bake for another 13 to 15 minutes, until a toothpick inserted in the center comes out clean or with just a few moist crumbs attached.

Cool the muffins in the tin for 5 minutes, then transfer to a wire rack to continue cooling. These muffins are best served warm

PRO TIP!

Baking the muffins at a high temperature at the beginning helps them rise quickly and get that dome-like structure you see in bakery-style muffins. Then we lower the heat to finish cooking the muffins all the way through.

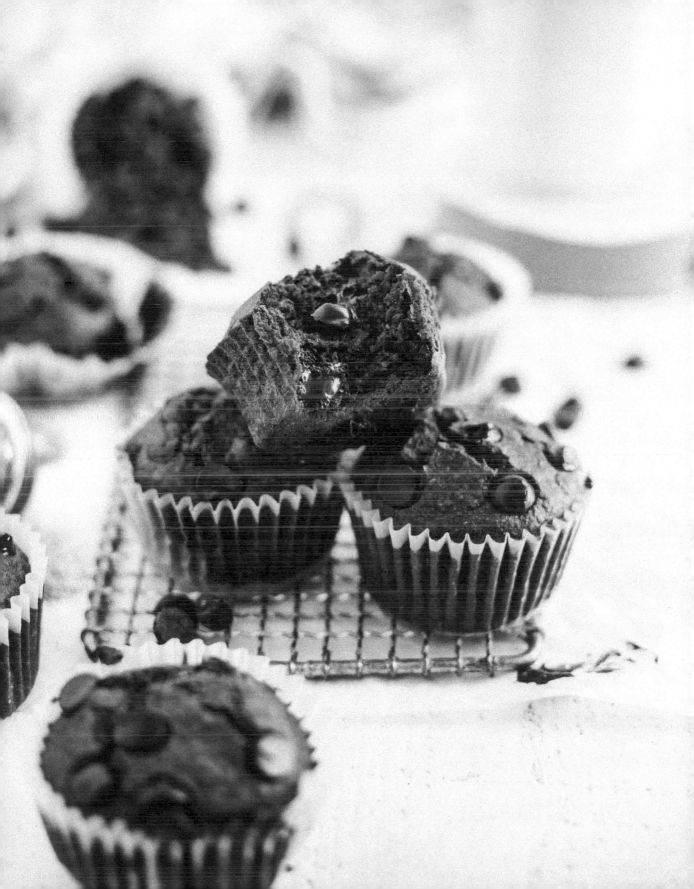

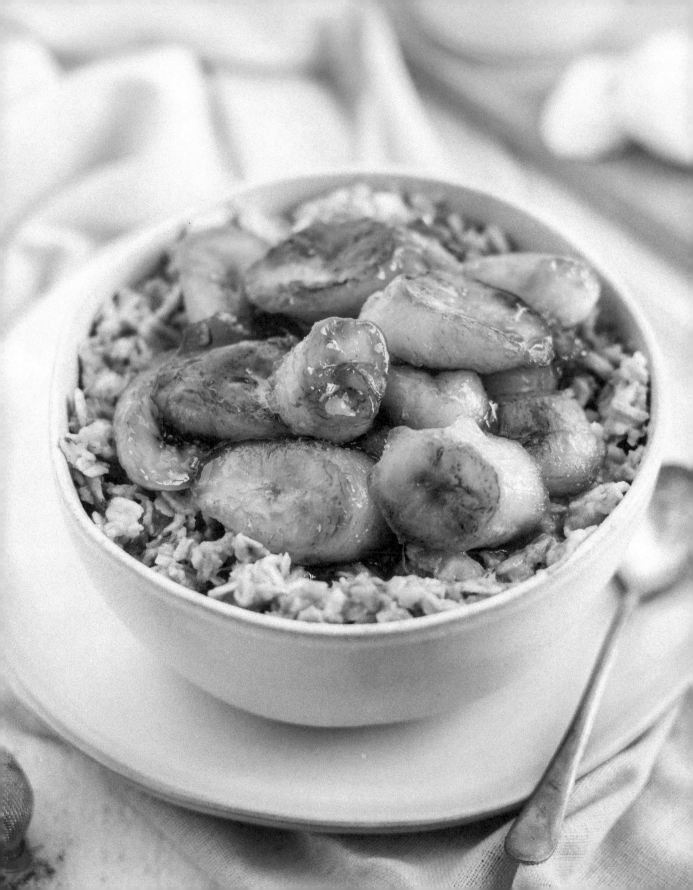

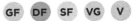

Caramelized Banana Oatmeal

Imagine having bananas Foster for breakfast! The natural sugars from the maple syrup and bananas caramelize in the pan and make a sweet topping to go with the healthy and fiber-filled oatmeal.

For the oatmeal:

1 cup (80 g) gluten-free rolled oats

1 medium ripe banana, mashed

1½ cups (355 ml) unsweetened vanilla nondairy milk, plus more for topping (optional)

2 teaspoons chia seeds

¼ teaspoon ground cinnamon

For the caramelized bananas:

2 tablespoons (28 g) coconut oil

2 tablespoons (40 g) pure maple syrup

2 small, ripe bananas, cut into ½-inch (1.25 cm) rounds

Nut butter, for topping (optional)

—

Yield | 2 servings

To make the oatmeal, combine the oats, mashed banana, milk, chia seeds, and cinnamon in a medium saucepan and bring to a simmer over medium-high heat. Cook for 5 to 8 minutes, stirring occasionally, until the milk is absorbed into the oats.

Meanwhile, to make the caramelized bananas, melt the coconut oil and maple syrup in a small cast-iron skillet over medium heat, stirring gently to combine. Layer the banana slices in the pan and cook for 2 to 3 minutes per side, until golden brown and caramelized.

Divide the oatmeal between 2 bowls and top with the caramelized bananas. Add more milk or a dollop of nut butter if desired.

Berry-Almond Smoothie Bowl

Start your day with a burst of berry flavor! This dairy-free smoothie bowl is full of antioxidants and inflammation-fighting berries, especially if you use blueberries, plus healthy fats from the nut butter to keep you full. Get creative with your healthy toppings and be sure to post it on Instagram—use the hashtag #WhatMollyMade so I can see your creation!

1½ cups (225 g) frozen berry mixture

½ cup (66 g) frozen cauliflower florets

1 banana, divided

3 tablespoons (45 g) almond butter

¼ cup (21 g) unsweetened coconut flakes

⅓ cup (79 ml) unsweetened vanilla nondairy milk

Chia seeds, fresh berries, muesli, granola, dark chocolate chips, and/or coconut flakes, for topping (optional)

—
Yield | 1 serving

Combine the berries, cauliflower, half of the banana, almond butter, coconut flakes, and milk in a blender and blend for 2 to 3 minutes, until creamy and smooth. The mixture will be thick, but this is what you want so you can eat it with a spoon. Spoon into a large bowl and top with the rest of the banana, sliced, and whatever other toppings you like. Enjoy immediately!

PRO TIP!

A high-powered blender like a Vitamix helps get this smoothie bowl really smooth and creamy! You can also use a food processor.

Egg and Bacon Cauliflower Bowls

This low-carb breakfast is packed with veggies and protein. Using the fat from the bacon to cook the veggies adds a depth of flavor you can't get anywhere else. This colorful bowl is full of vitamins and nutrients your body needs to fight inflammation.

3 strips nitrate-free, sugar-free bacon (about 3 ounces/85 g total)

1 small yellow onion, diced

1 bell pepper (any color), seeded and diced

2 cups (60 g) baby spinach

3 cups (321 g) riced cauliflower

2 teaspoons coconut aminos

¼ teaspoon salt

⅛ teaspoon black pepper

4 large eggs

Chopped scallions, for garnish (optional)

—

Yield | 4 servings

Heat a large skillet over medium- high heat. Add the bacon and cook until crisp, about 3 minutes per side. Transfer the cooked bacon to paper towels to cool, then crumble.

Drain off all but 1 to 2 tablespoons (15 to 30 ml) of bacon fat from the skillet. Add the onion and bell pepper and cook over medium heat until both are soft and the onion is translucent, 3 to 5 minutes. Add the spinach and cover for 30 to 60 seconds to wilt. Add the riced cauliflower, crumbled bacon, coconut aminos, salt, and pepper and stir well.

Create 4 wells in the cauliflower mixture with the back of a spoon. Crack an egg into each well and cover the skillet. Cook for 2 to 3 minutes for runny eggs, or longer for your desired doneness. Garnish with chopped scallions.

> **PRO TIP!**
>
> You can make this recipe ahead of time by cooking the cauliflower hash and storing it in an airtight container in the fridge. When you're ready to eat, reheat the hash in the skillet, cook the eggs as instructed, and enjoy!

Sweet Potato Waffle Breakfast Sandwich

Did you know sweet potatoes can be turned into waffles? Simply shred, mix, and cook in a waffle iron for a crispy, anti-inflammatory waffle. When you bite into this sandwich, the runny egg oozes out and the spicy sriracha sauce adds the perfect kick. This one will impress all your friends and family!

For the sweet potato waffles:

2 large eggs

1 large sweet potato, scrubbed and grated

½ teaspoon garlic powder

¼ teaspoon salt

⅛ teaspoon paprika

Nonstick cooking spray

For the egg sandwich:

4 strips nitrate-free, sugar-free bacon (about 4 ounces/113 g total)

3 cups (90 g) kale, stemmed and chopped

¼ teaspoon salt

⅛ teaspoon black pepper

2 large eggs

½ avocado, peeled, pitted, and sliced

For the sriracha aioli:

¼ cup (60 g) paleo mayonnaise

2 teaspoons sriracha, or more to taste

—

Yield | 2 sandwiches

To make the sweet potato waffles, preheat a waffle iron. In a medium bowl, mix the eggs, shredded sweet potato, garlic powder, salt, and paprika. Once the waffle iron is fully heated, spray both sides with nonstick cooking spray. Add the mixture to the waffle iron, spreading to each quadrant. Press the waffle iron lid down gently and cook for 5 to 7 minutes, until the edges are crispy and the middle is set. The waffles should turn lightly golden and hold together well.

To make the sandwich filling, while the waffles are cooking, heat a large skillet over medium-high heat and add the bacon. Cook until crisp, about 3 minutes per side. Transfer the bacon to paper towels to absorb the grease. Drain off all but 2 to 3 tablespoons (28 to 42 g) of bacon fat from the skillet.

Add the chopped kale, salt, and pepper and cook over medium heat, stirring, until crisp, 3 to 4 minutes. Move the kale to the sides of the pan and crack the eggs in the center. Cook until the egg whites look set, about 2 minutes, then flip and cook on the other side for 1 minute. The egg yolks should still be soft. Remove the pan from the heat.

To make the sriracha aioli, whisk together the mayo and sriracha in a small bowl.

When the sweet potato waffles are done, divide the kale between two waffles. Add a fried egg, 2 slices of cooked bacon, and sliced avocado on top of each waffle. Finish with the sriracha aioli, then close each sandwich with the remaining sweet potato waffles. Enjoy immediately with your hands or a fork.

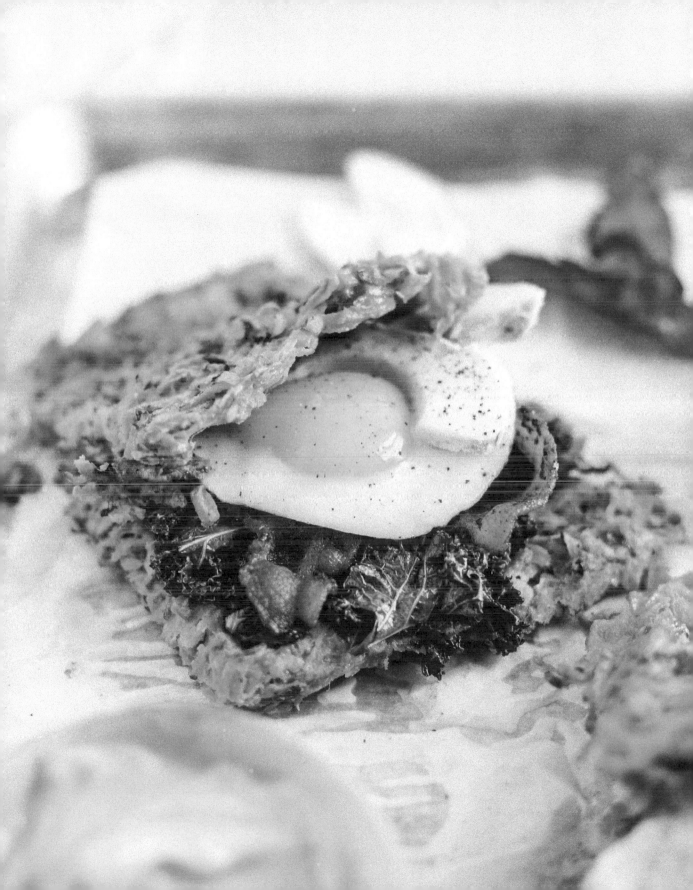

Rosemary-Sage Turkey Sausage Patties with Sweet Potatoes

With minimal cleaning and prep required, this recipe makes a great weekend brunch or easy meal to prep for the week. Sweet potatoes are high in vitamin A and beta-carotene—a powerful antioxidant.

For the sweet potatoes:

2 large sweet potatoes, scrubbed and cut into ½-inch (1.25 cm) cubes

2 tablespoons (30 ml) olive oil

1½ teaspoons garlic powder

1 teaspoon paprika

½ teaspoon onion powder

½ teaspoon salt

⅛ teaspoon black pepper

For the sausage patties:

1 pound (454 g) ground turkey

2 tablespoons (40 g) pure maple syrup

1 tablespoon (4 g) chopped fresh sage

1½ teaspoons chopped fresh rosemary

¾ teaspoon salt

½ teaspoon crushed fennel seeds

¼ teaspoon black pepper

Pinch ground nutmeg (optional)

—
Yield | 12 lettuce wraps

Preheat the oven to 400°F (200°C). Line a rimmed baking sheet with a silicone baking mat or aluminum foil.

To make the sweet potatoes, on the prepared baking sheet, toss the sweet potatoes with the olive oil, garlic powder, paprika, onion powder, salt, and pepper. Spread out in a single layer. Roast for 15 minutes.

To make the sausage patties, combine all the patty ingredients in a medium bowl. Using a heaping tablespoon (15 g), scoop the sausage mixture and shape into 2-inch (5 cm) balls, then flatten into patties. You should have about 12 patties.

When the sweet potatoes have roasted for 15 minutes, stir them and push them to one side to make room for the sausage patties. Arrange the patties about 1 inch (2.5 cm) apart on the baking sheet. Roast for 10 minutes.

Remove the baking sheet from the oven and turn the oven to broil. Flip the sausage patties and stir the potatoes one more time. Broil for 2 to 3 minutes, until the sausage and potatoes are slightly browned and the patties reach an internal temperature of 160°F (70°C). Enjoy immediately.

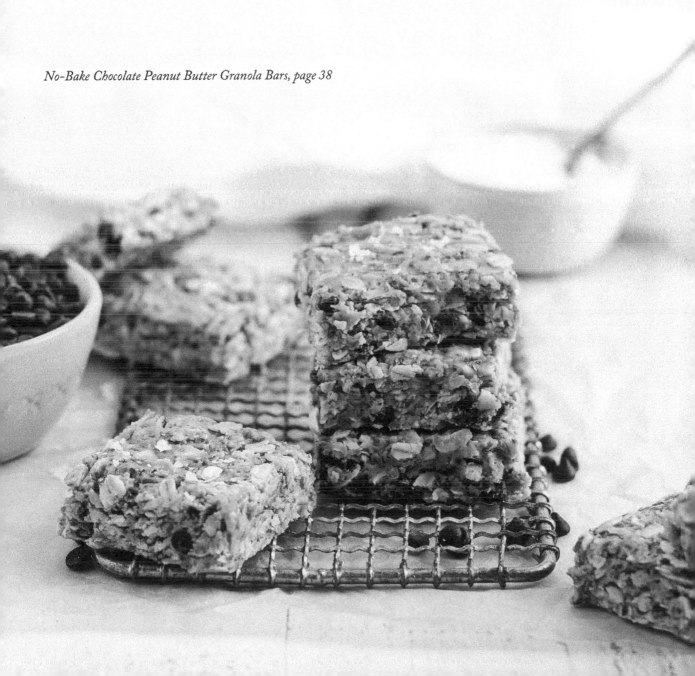

CHAPTER THREE

Dips, Spreads, and Snacks

No-Bake Chocolate Peanut Butter Granola Bars, page 38

Spicy Chicken Thai-Inspired Lettuce Wraps

Boston lettuce holds a spicy, sweet, crunchy Asian fusion filling in these lettuce wraps. The filling makes great leftovers, so pack a bowl with some extra lettuce for a lunch you'll look forward to.

For the peanut sauce:

½ cup (130 g) creamy natural peanut butter

¼ cup (63 g) coconut aminos

Juice of 1 lime

1 tablespoon (20 g) chile paste

1 tablespoon (20 g) pure maple syrup or raw honey

1 tablespoon (15 ml) toasted sesame oil

2 teaspoons minced garlic

For the lettuce wraps:

1 pound (454 g) ground chicken

¼ cup (35 g) chopped peanuts, plus more for garnish

2 tablespoons (30 ml) toasted sesame oil

12 Boston lettuce or butter lettuce leaves

¼ cup (23 g) shredded carrots

¼ cup (23 g) thinly sliced red cabbage

2 to 3 teaspoons sesame seeds, for topping

Chopped fresh cilantro and chopped scallion, for garnish

—

Yield | 12 lettuce wraps

To make the peanut sauce, heat the peanut butter in a microwave-safe bowl on high for 30 seconds, or until smooth enough to pour. Add the rest of the sauce ingredients and whisk well.

To make the lettuce wraps, pour three-quarters of the peanut sauce into a bowl and add the ground chicken and chopped peanuts. Stir to combine, cover, and refrigerate for 15 minutes to marinate.

Heat the sesame oil in a medium skillet over medium-high heat. Add the marinated chicken and cook, stirring frequently to break up the meat, until cooked through, 2 to 3 minutes.

Spoon the chicken mixture into the lettuce leaves and top each with shredded carrot, sliced cabbage, sesame seeds, cilantro, scallions, and more chopped peanuts. Drizzle with the remaining peanut sauce and serve.

PRO TIP!

If you aren't a huge fan of spice, just omit the chile paste. This will give you a mild flavor that's just as delicious!

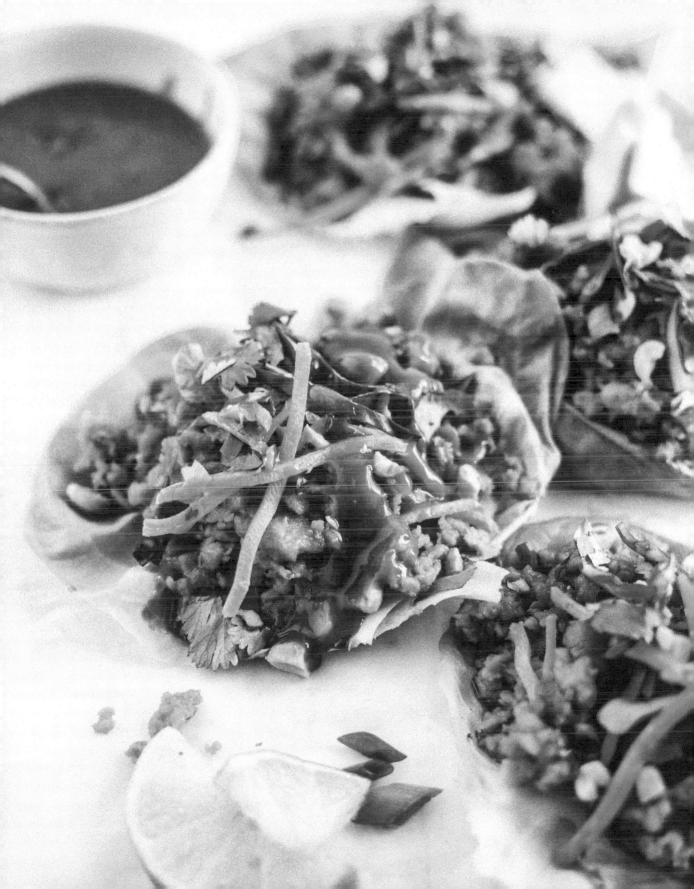

Buffalo Cauliflower with Ranch

Fool your friends (in a good way!) with these Buffalo "wings." The batter coats the veggies and crisps in the oven within minutes. I love how the honey from the sauce sweetens it and caramelizes a bit when it cooks. If you're anything like me, you'll crave this not only on weekends for parties but also for a great Meatless Monday dinner!

For the cauliflower:

1 cup (112 g) almond flour

½ cup (64 g) tapioca flour

2 teaspoons garlic powder

1 teaspoon paprika

1 teaspoon salt

½ teaspoon black pepper

¾ cup (175 ml) unsweetened nondairy milk

4 cups (400 g) cauliflower florets

For the Buffalo sauce:

¾ cup (175 ml) hot sauce, such as Frank's RedHot sauce

3 tablespoons (60 g) raw honey

Dairy-free ranch dressing for serving

Carrot and celery sticks, for serving

—
Yield | 6 servings

Preheat the oven to 350°F (180°C). Line a rimmed baking sheet with a silicone baking mat or parchment paper.

To make the cauliflower, in a large mixing bowl, whisk together the almond flour, tapioca flour, garlic powder, paprika, salt, and pepper. Add the milk and whisk to form a batter.

Dip each cauliflower floret into the batter, turning until it's completely coated, then place in a single layer on the prepared baking sheet. Bake for 20 minutes, turn gently, and bake for another 10 minutes, or until golden brown.

To make the Buffalo sauce, in a large bowl, mix the hot sauce and honey. Add the baked cauliflower to the sauce and stir gently to coat, being careful not to remove the breading from the cauliflower. Dump the coated cauliflower back onto the same baking sheet, spread into a single layer, and bake for another 10 minutes to absorb all the sauce.

Serve right away with ranch dressing and carrots and celery.

Peanut Butter Dates with Cocoa Nibs

This may sound like an unlikely combo, but the sweet dates, salty peanut butter, and crunch from the cocoa nibs create a bite full of carbs and fat that you'll never forget.

12 Medjool dates

¼ cup (65 g) natural peanut butter

1 ounce (28 g) cocoa nibs

Sea salt, to taste

—

Yield | 12 dates

Make a long lengthwise slit down the center of each date. Remove the pits. Spoon 1 teaspoon peanut butter into the cavity where the pit was. Sprinkle with the cocoa nibs and sea salt.

PRO TIP!

The peak season for dates is mid-autumn through mid-winter, but you can find them in the local grocery store year-round. Medjool dates are extra large—perfect for stuffing!

Snickerdoodle Energy Bites

If you love snickerdoodle cookies, these sweet bite-size snacks will get you through the afternoon hump. I also enjoy them as a bedtime snack!

For the energy bites:

1½ cups (120 g) gluten-free oat flour

¾ cup (180 g) cashew butter

⅓ cup (115 g) raw honey

¼ cup (56 g) coconut oil, at room temperature

½ teaspoon pure vanilla extract

1½ teaspoons ground cinnamon

¼ teaspoon sea salt

For the cinnamon-sugar coating (optional):

¼ cup (50 g) coconut sugar

1 teaspoon ground cinnamon

—

Yield | 14 bites

To make the energy bites, combine all the energy bite ingredients in a food processor and blend on high until completely incorporated, about 1 minute. If the mixture is too wet, add more oat flour, 1 tablespoon (5 g) at a time. If it's too dry, add more honey and nut butter. Form the dough into 1½-inch (4 cm) balls.

If you're making the cinnamon-sugar coating, mix those ingredients together in a small bowl, then roll the balls in the cinnamon-sugar. Place on a rimmed baking sheet. Refrigerate for at least 30 minutes before serving. Store in an airtight container in the refrigerator.

No-Bake Chocolate Peanut Butter Granola Bars

A grab-and-go breakfast and snack is always a good recipe to have in your repertoire. Sometimes I'm rushing out the door with my coffee in hand and have to run back inside to grab one of these granola bars. As a new mom, I love having simple, healthy snacks like this on hand.

⅔ cup (97 g) raw, unsalted cashews

⅓ cup (48 g) raw, unsalted pecans

1 cup (260 g) creamy natural peanut butter

½ cup (170 g) raw honey

1½ cups (120 g) gluten-free rolled oats

⅓ cup (56 g) ground flaxseed

½ cup (88 g) mini dairy-free chocolate chips

—
Yield | 16 squares

Line an 8-inch (20 cm) square baking pan with parchment paper. Leave extra on the sides to use as handles for easily removing the bars from the pan when they're done.

Combine the cashews and pecans in a food processor and pulse a few times to crush the nuts.

In a large microwave-safe bowl, microwave the peanut butter on high for 30 seconds. Add the honey and mix together quickly, then add the crushed nuts, oats, flaxseed, and chocolate chips. Use a silicone spatula to mix everything together, making sure everything is fully coated.

Pour the mixture into the prepared baking pan and press down firmly with the spatula until the top is completely even. Refrigerate for at least 45 minutes, then cutinto 16 squares.

PRO TIP!

Make a double batch of these and store in an airtight container in the freezer for up to 6 months.

Two-Ingredient Grain-Free Tortillas

Say goodbye to tortillas that break and fall apart. Fry these sturdy tortillas for a few minutes, then fill them with your favorite ingredients. You'll love using them for tacos, roll-ups for lunch, and even a breakfast wrap with almond butter and granola—or a sweet treat with melted coconut oil, sugar, and cinnamon.

2 large (6 ounces, or 170 g) sweet potatoes, peeled and cut into 1-inch (2.5 cm) pieces

1 cup (137 g) cassava flour, plus more for dusting

1 to 2 tablespoons (15 to 30 ml) olive oil

—
Yield | 10 tortillas

Put the sweet potatoes in a large pot and cover with water. Cover and bring to a boil over medium-high heat. Boil for 3 to 5 minutes, until the potatoes are fork-tender. Drain the sweet potatoes and transfer to a food processor. Add the cassava flour and blend on high for 1 to 2 minutes, until the mixture starts to pull away from the sides of the bowl.

Dust a clean, dry work surface and a rolling pin with additional cassava flour. Divide the sweet potato dough into 10 equal pieces and roll each into a disk about ¼ inch (6 mm) thick.

Heat the olive oil in a large skillet over medium heat. One at a time, heat the tortillas, turning halfway through, for 3 minutes, or until lightly golden brown and starting to bubble. Transfer to a paper towel–lined plate and repeat until all of the tortillas are cooked.

PRO TIP!

I like to make a large batch of these sweet potato tortillas at once. They reheat well, so you can meal prep in advance. Store in an airtight container in the refrigerator for up to 1 week or in the freezer for up to 3 months. Thaw overnight in the refrigerator before using.

Salted Vanilla-Maple Cashew Butter

With just a few ingredients, you can make this sweet and salty spread. Roasting the cashews first gives them a toasted flavor you can't find in nut butters at the store. I love this on Sweet Potato Toast 4 Ways (page 20) with sliced apples and cinnamon, and on oatmeal or pancakes.

3 cups (435 g) raw, unsalted cashews

1 tablespoon (15 ml) pure vanilla extract

1 tablespoon (20 g) pure maple syrup

2 teaspoons coconut oil

1 teaspoon sea salt

Flaky sea salt, for topping (optional)

—

Yield | 6 to 8 servings

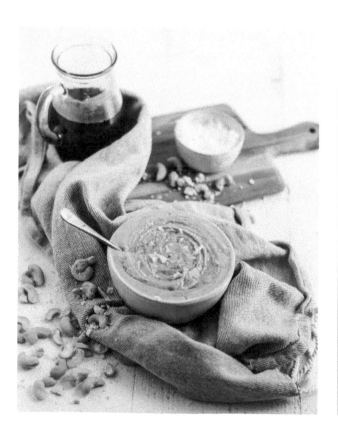

Preheat the oven to 350°F (180°C). Line a rimmed baking sheet with parchment paper or aluminum foil.

Spread the cashews on the prepared baking sheet and bake for 10 to 12 minutes, until fragrant and lightly toasted. Let cool for 5 minutes.

Transfer the toasted cashews to a food processor or high-powered blender. Blend until the cashews are broken down into a smooth, spreadable butter with no clumps, 10 to 15 minutes in a food processor or 3 to 5 minutes in a high-powered blender. Add the vanilla, maple syrup, coconut oil, and salt and blend for another 1 to 2 minutes to combine.

Transfer to an airtight container and top with flaky sea salt, if desired. Store at room temperature for up to 3 weeks.

PRO TIP!

Don't give up on the processing! Blending time will vary, and may take up to 20 minutes, depending on the strength of your blender or food processor.

Kale, Chorizo, and Artichoke Dip

Your guests will never guess that this dip is dairy-free. By making the base with mayo and coconut cream, you get a thick, creamy texture. The nutritional yeast adds a cheesy flavor that contrasts perfectly with the spicy chorizo. For this recipe you want Mexican-style fresh (raw) chorizo, rather than Spanish-style dry (cured) chorizo.

Nonstick cooking spray

8 ounces (227 g) fresh chorizo (no sugar added)

1 medium yellow onion, diced

4 garlic cloves, minced

8 ounces (227 g) kale, stemmed and roughly chopped

1 (14-ounce/397 g) can artichoke hearts, drained and roughly chopped

Salt and black pepper, to taste

For the cream mixture:

1 cup (225 g) paleo mayonnaise

1 cup (230 g) canned coconut cream

⅓ cup (33 g) nutritional yeast

1 tablespoon (15 ml) lemon juice

2 tablespoons (16 g) tapioca flour

Salt and black pepper, to taste

Sweet potato chips, carrot sticks, celery sticks, or almond flour crackers, for serving

—
Yield | 6 to 8 servings

Preheat the oven to 400°F (200°C). Spray an 8-inch (20 cm) square baking pan or small casserole dish with nonstick cooking spray.

Heat a large skillet over medium heat. Add the chorizo and cook, stirring often to break up the meat, for about 5 minutes, or until the chorizo is browned. Transfer the chorizo to paper towels. Drain off all about 1 tablespoon (15 ml) of fat from the pan.

Add the onion and cook until soft and translucent, 2 to 3 minutes. Add the garlic and continue to cook until fragrant, another 1 to 2 minutes. Add the kale and sauté until wilted, about 5 minutes. It will seem like a lot of kale, but it will cook down. Return the cooked chorizo to the pan, add the artichokes, and cook for another 1 to 2 minutes to heat through. Season with salt and pepper and mix well. Remove the pan from the heat.

To make the cream mixture, combine all the ingredients in a large bowl and mix using a handheld mixer or whisk.

Add the kale mixture to the cream mixture, discarding any extra liquid in the bottom of the pan. Mix well until fully combined. Transfer the dip to the prepared baking pan.

Bake for 25 to 30 minutes, until heated through and bubbling around the edges. Let the dip cool for 5 to 10 minutes, then serve with your favorite dippers.

PRO TIP!

You can buy a can of coconut cream or use the coconut cream from the top of a can of full-fat coconut milk.

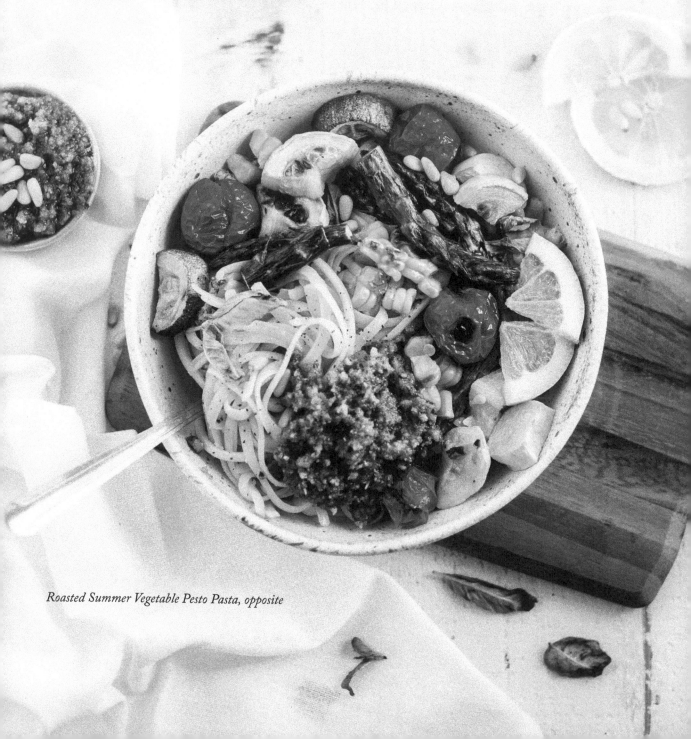

CHAPTER FOUR

Pasta and Grains

Roasted Summer Vegetable Pesto Pasta, opposite

Roasted Summer Vegetable Pesto Pasta

Ever browse the farmers' market and think you'd love to buy all the veggies but have no idea what to make with them? This pesto pasta is the answer. If you pick up another veggie in season, feel free to swap it out! You can't go wrong with any roasted veggie, and they're all great for fighting inflammation.

For the pasta:

2 ears corn, shucked

2 cups (180 g) cherry tomatoes

2 cups (142 g) chopped asparagus

1 medium zucchini, halved lengthwise and sliced crosswise

1 medium yellow squash, halved lengthwise and sliced crosswise

2 tablespoons (30 ml) olive oil

1 teaspoon sea salt

8 ounces (226 g) gluten-free linguine (chickpea or brown rice pasta)

For the pesto:

1 cup (135 g) pine nuts

1½ cups (60 g) tightly packed fresh basil leaves

1 garlic clove, peeled

3 tablespoons (15 g) nutritional yeast

¼ cup (59 ml) light-tasting olive oil

Juice of 1 lemon

½ teaspoon salt

—
Yield | 4 servings

Preheat the oven to 425°F (220°C). Line a rimmed baking sheet with aluminum foil.

To make the pasta, stand each ear of corn on its end in a shallow dish and cut the kernels off the cob.

Spread out the corn, tomatoes, asparagus, zucchini, and squash in a single layer on the prepared baking sheet. Drizzle with the olive oil and sprinkle with the sea salt. Roast for 25 minutes, or until fork-tender. Remove the baking sheet from the oven and turn the oven to broil. Stir the veggies, then broil for 2 to 3 minutes, until browned.

While the veggies roast, cook the pasta according to the package directions until al dente. Drain the pasta and return it to the stockpot.

To make the pesto, combine all the pesto ingredients in a food processor and blend on high until smooth.

Add the roasted vegetables to the pasta and stir well. Serve in bowls and top each serving with a large scoop of pesto. You can also mix the pesto with the veggies and pasta in the pot to coat.

ADD IT!

Looking for a little extra protein to add to this recipe? Fry an egg and place it right on top of the bowl of pasta and veggies. The runny yolk is the perfect addition to the pesto sauce.

Sweet Potato Gnocchi with Sausage and Cream Sauce

Keep this recipe in your pocket when you're trying to impress! It's great for date nights or special family occasions. No one will know this comforting meal is gluten- and dairy-free. The beta-carotene from the sweet potatoes adds powerful antioxidants to your meal, along with spinach, one of the best-known anti-inflammatory foods.

For the gnocchi:

4 pounds (1815 g) sweet potatoes (about 4 large potatoes), peeled and cut into chunks

1 cup (137 g) cassava flour, plus more as needed

Pinch salt

1½ tablespoons (22 ml) olive oil

For the sauce:

2 tablespoons (30 ml) olive oil

½ yellow onion, chopped

3 large garlic cloves, minced

12 ounces (340 g) sugar-free andouille sausage, sliced into ½-inch (1.3 cm) pieces on the bias

1 cup (70 g) sliced cremini mushrooms

1 (13.5-ounce/383 g) can full-fat coconut milk

1 tablespoon (8 g) tapioca flour

1 tablespoon (4 g) chopped fresh rosemary

1 tablespoon (4 g) chopped fresh thyme

½ teaspoon sea salt

¼ teaspoon black pepper

2 cups (60 g) fresh baby spinach

—

Yield | 6 servings

PRO TIP!

Make a double batch of gnocchi and put half in your freezer for an easy weeknight meal. Once they're cut, place on a baking sheet and put in the freezer for 30 minutes, then transfer to a resealable plastic bag and store in the freezer. When ready to cook, add the frozen gnocchi right to the boiling water!

To make the gnocchi, put the sweet potatoes in a large stockpot and cover with water. Bring the water to a boil over high heat and cook for 10 to 15 minutes, until the potatoes are easily pierced with a fork. Drain the potatoes and transfer to a large bowl. Reserve the stockpot.

Add the cassava flour to the sweet potatoes and stir together with a wooden spoon. When it gets difficult to stir, switch to using your hands. Mix and knead until the dough starts to form a ball. If the dough is too wet, add cassava flour, 1 tablespoon (8 g) at a time, until the dough forms a ball and isn't very sticky.

Dust a clean, dry work surface with cassava flour. Divide the dough into 4 equal parts. Roll out one part into a long rope, about 1 inch (2.5 cm) in diameter. Starting at one end, cut the dough into 1-inch (2.5 cm) pieces. Repeat with the remaining dough. If you like, make mini fork marks with the back of the fork on each gnocchi.

Fill the same stockpot about halfway with fresh water. Add a pinch of salt and bring to a boil over high heat. While it's heating, place a rimmed baking sheet next to the stove to set the cooked gnocchi on. Add one-fourth of the gnocchi to the boiling water. The gnocchi will sink to the bottom. Once they float to the top,

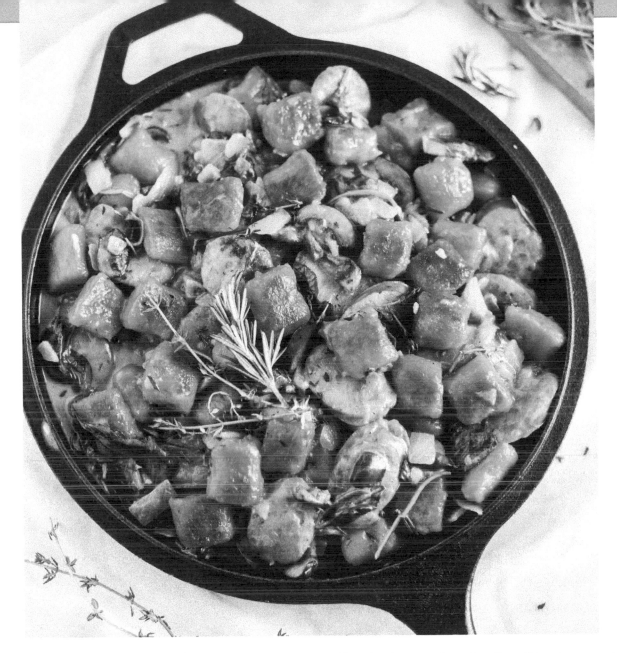

remove them with a slotted spoon and place on the baking sheet. Repeat the process with the remaining gnocchi.

Heat the olive oil in a large skillet over medium heat. Add the gnocchi and sear on one side for 1 to 2 minutes, until golden brown. Flip and sear the other side. Transfer the gnocchi to a plate.

To make the sauce, heat the olive oil in a large sauté pan over medium-high heat. Add the onion and garlic and cook until translucent, 2 to 3 minutes. Add the sausage, mushrooms, coconut milk, tapioca flour, rosemary, thyme, salt, and pepper and bring the sauce to a boil. Cook for 2 to 3 minutes to thicken. Stir in the spinach and cook until it wilts, then add the gnocchi and stir to coat.

One-Pot Taco Pasta

Taco Tuesday, pasta style! You only need one pot and less than 20 minutes to have an anti-inflammatory dinner on the table. The pasta cooks in the same pan as the meat and gives the noodles an extra boost of taco flavor without the need for another pot or strainer.

2 tablespoons (30 ml) olive oil

1 medium yellow onion, diced

2 garlic cloves, minced

1 pound (454 g) ground beef

1 (1-ounce/28 g) packet sugar-free taco seasoning

2½ cups (591 ml) water, divided

1 cup (260 g) mild salsa

12 ounces (340 g) gluten-free rotini (chickpea or brown rice pasta)

1 cup (172 g) rinsed and drained canned black beans

1 cup (225 g) drained canned corn

1 cup (150 g) cherry tomatoes, chopped

1 avocado, peeled, pitted, and diced

Lime juice and chopped fresh cilantro, for topping (optional)

—
Yield | 6 servings

Heat the olive oil in a large pot or Dutch oven over high heat. Add the onion, garlic, and beef and cook, breaking up the meat, for about 3 minutes, until completely browned.

Add the packet of taco seasoning and ½ cup (118 ml) of the water and stir well. Add the remaining 2 cups (473 ml) water, salsa, and uncooked rotini and stir. Cover, reduce the heat to medium-low, and cook for about 15 minutes, until the pasta is cooked al dente and the liquid is absorbed.

Add the black beans, corn, cherry tomatoes, and avocado. Top with a squeeze of lime juice and cilantro if desired.

Southwest Stuffed Peppers

Stuffed peppers are part of traditional Spanish cuisine, but we're giving them a Southwest flair with the addition of black beans, corn, and spices like cumin and chili powder. Everyone loves this dish, and it just so happens to be gluten- and dairy-free.

½ cup (98 g) long-grain white or brown rice

1¼ cups (296 ml) hot water

1 tablespoon (14 g) coconut oil

1 medium yellow onion, diced

3 garlic cloves, minced

1 pound (454 g) ground beef or ground turkey

1 cup (245 g) tomato sauce

1 (15-ounce/425 g) can yellow corn, drained

1 (15-ounce/432 g) can black beans, rinsed and drained

1 (4-ounce/113 g) can roasted green chiles, drained

2 cups (134 g) chopped kale

2 tablespoons (15 g) chili powder

2 to 2½ teaspoons ground cumin

1 teaspoon sea salt

½ teaspoon black pepper

7 large bell peppers (any color)

Chopped avocado, chopped fresh cilantro, salsa, and chopped red onion, for topping (optional)

—
Yield | 7 stuffed peppers

Preheat the oven to 350°F (180°C).

Combine the rice and hot water in a 9-inch (23 cm) square casserole dish or baking pan. Cover tightly with aluminum foil and bake for 25 minutes, or until all the water is absorbed.

While the rice is cooking, melt the coconut oil in a large skillet over medium-high heat. Add the onion and cook until soft and translucent, 2 to 3 minutes. Add the garlic and cook for another 1 to 2 minutes, until fragrant. Add the ground beef and cook, stirring occasionally, until browned and no pink remains, 3 to 5 minutes.

Add the tomato sauce, corn, black beans, chiles, and kale and cook, stirring frequently, until the kale is wilted, 2 to 3 minutes. Add the chili powder, cumin, salt, and pepper and stir well to combine. Remove from the heat. When the rice is done, add the rice to the ground beef mixture and stir well.

Slice the tops off the bell peppers and remove the seeds and ribs inside. Stand the bell peppers in the same dish the rice was in. Using a large spoon, evenly divide the beef mixture into the peppers until filled to the top. Cover with foil and bake for 45 minutes. Remove from the oven and top with cilantro, avocado, salsa, and red onion, if desired.

PRO TIP!

You can make the rice on the stovetop if you prefer, but I love baking it in the oven while the filling is cooking. It saves a dish to clean and it turns out light and fluffy every time.

Blackened Chicken Tacos with Cilantro-Lime Rice

Wait until you add this recipe to your Taco Tuesday lineup! The hearty cilantro-lime rice makes these tacos a full meal without the need for any sides. If you like, you can even make burrito bowls instead of tacos. The spices from the blackened seasoning are a great example of how anti-inflammatory ingredients can add so much flavor to a dish.

For the cilantro-lime rice:

1 teaspoon olive oil

⅓ cup (55 g) finely chopped onion

2 garlic cloves, minced

½ teaspoon sea salt

½ cup (98 g) long-grain white rice

1 cup (237 ml) vegetable broth

Juice of ½ lime

½ cup (32 g) finely chopped fresh cilantro

For the blackened chicken:

1 teaspoon smoked paprika

1 teaspoon ground cumin

1 teaspoon garlic powder

½ teaspoon dried oregano

½ teaspoon onion powder

½ teaspoon salt

¼ teaspoon black pepper

¼ teaspoon cayenne pepper

1½ pounds (680 g) boneless, skinless chicken breasts

1 tablespoon (15 ml) olive oil

For the pineapple salsa:

3 cups (495 g) drained crushed canned pineapple

½ small red bell pepper, seeded and chopped

½ cup (80 g) chopped red onion

¼ cup (16 g) finely chopped fresh cilantro

Juice of 1 lime

½ teaspoon salt

For serving:

8 Two-Ingredient Grain-Free Tortillas (page 39) or store-bought grain-free tortillas

Chopped avocado and chopped fresh cilantro, for topping

—

Yield | 4 servings

To make the rice, heat the olive oil in a large sauté pan over medium-high heat until it starts to ripple. Add the onion and cook for 2 to 3 minutes, until it starts to soften and become translucent. Add the garlic, salt, and rice and stir to toast for 1 to 2 minutes. Add the vegetable broth, cover, turn the heat up to high, and bring the mixture to a boil. Turn the heat down to low and allow to simmer, covered, for 15 to 20 minutes, until the rice absorbs all the liquid. Do not stir the rice while it cooks, or it can become sticky.

To make the chicken, while the rice is cooking, combine all the blackened chicken spices in a small bowl. Pat the chicken breasts dry with a paper towel and sprinkle both sides with the spice mixture, rubbing it in with your fingers.

Heat the olive oil in another sauté pan over medium heat until it starts to ripple. Add the chicken breasts, cover, and cook without moving them for 6 to 8 minutes on each side, to create a blackened crust. The chicken should reach an internal temperature of 165°F (74°C). Transfer the chicken to a cutting board and allow to rest for 5 to 10 minutes.

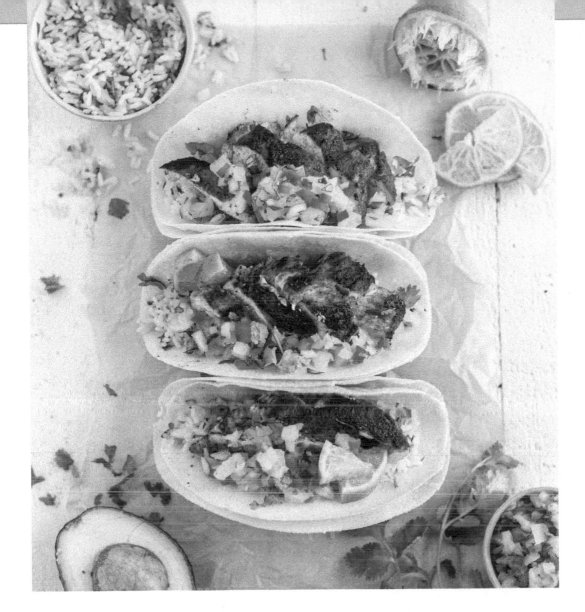

To make the salsa, while the chicken is resting, combine all the pineapple salsa ingredients in a medium bowl and stir well.

When the rice is done cooking, immediately add the lime juice and cilantro and stir well. Slice the chicken into strips.

Assemble the tacos by filling the tortillas with rice, chicken strips, and pineapple salsa. Top with avocado and extra cilantro, if desired.

PRO TIP!

A cast-iron skillet works best for this recipe because it distributes the heat and cooks the chicken evenly. It also creates the crust that is so famously associated with blackened chicken.

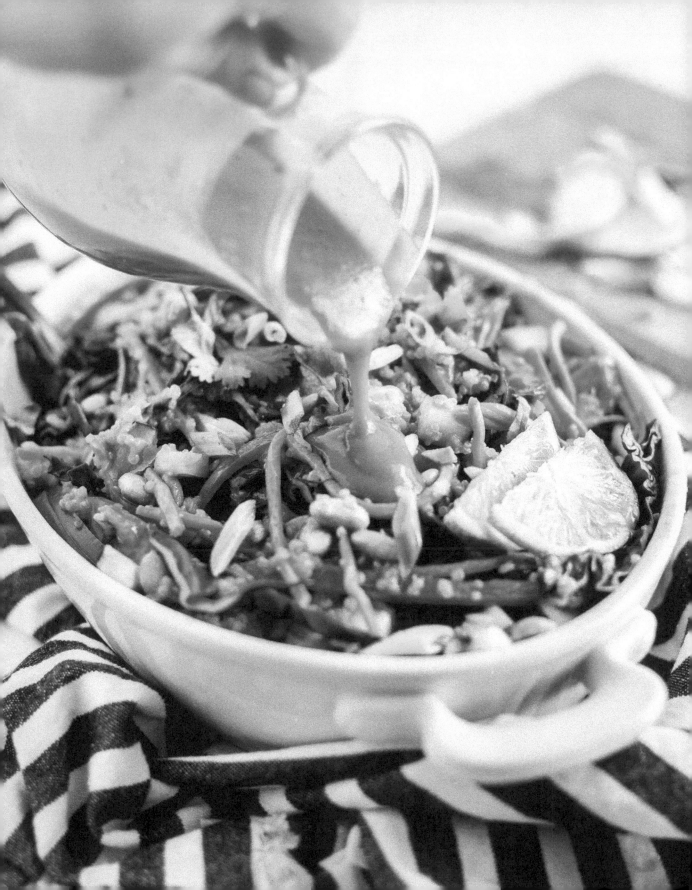

Crunchy Thai-Inspired Quinoa Salad with Peanut Dressing

This recipe is packed with flavor (hello, red chile paste!), vibrant colors, and plenty of vitamins and nutrients to help fight inflammation. We love to make this on a Sunday and throw several portions in meal prep containers to take for lunch throughout the week. You can add fresh herbs to brighten it up—my favorites are cilantro and Thai basil.

For the quinoa salad:

1½ cups (260 g) quinoa

1 cup (130 g) frozen edamame

2 cups (140 g) shredded purple cabbage

1 red or yellow bell pepper, seeded and thinly sliced

1 cup (110 g) shredded carrots

1 small cucumber, diced

½ cup (75 g) peanuts or cashews

½ cup (35 g) scallions, thinly sliced on the bias

Fresh Thai basil or cilantro, for garnish

Juice of 1 lime

For the peanut dressing:

⅓ cup (87 g) natural peanut butter, melted

¼ cup (63 g) coconut aminos

¼ cup (59 ml) rice vinegar

¼ cup (59 ml) toasted sesame oil

1 tablespoon (20 g) pure maple syrup or raw honey

1 teaspoon red chili paste

1 garlic clove, peeled

1 teaspoon fresh grated ginger

—

Yield | 6 servings

To make the quinoa salad, cook the quinoa and frozen edamame according to the package directions.

To make the peanut dressing, combine all the ingredients in a food processor and blend for 30 to 60 seconds, until smooth and creamy.

Assemble the salad by pouring the cooked quinoa into a large bowl. Top with the edamame, cabbage, bell pepper, carrots, cucumber, and nuts and drizzle with the peanut dressing. Toss to coat, then top with the scallions, herbs, and lime juice.

PRO TIP!

You can also assemble individual salads for guests or meal prep. Just divide everything evenly into 6 small bowls.

Mediterranean Quinoa Bowls with Roasted Red Pepper Sauce

This recipe is full of veggies, healthy fats, and whole grains. It's rich in omega-3 fatty acids that help fight inflammation and fill you up at the same time.

For the bowls:

2 cups (475 ml) vegetable or chicken broth

1 cup (173 g) quinoa

1 cup (240) rinsed and drained canned chickpeas

1 cup (150 g) grape tomatoes, halved

1 cup (100 g) kalamata olives

1 cup (135 g) diced cucumber

½ cup (80 g) diced red onion

2 tablespoons (30 ml) olive oil

Juice of ½ lemon

1 teaspoon dried oregano

1 teaspoon dried rosemary

¼ teaspoon dried dill

¼ teaspoon salt

¼ teaspoon black pepper

For the roasted red pepper sauce:

1 (12-ounce/340 g)jar roasted red peppers, drained

¼ cup (59 ml) light olive oil

¼ teaspoon salt

Juice of ½ lemon

2 garlic cloves, peeled

½ small shallot, roughly chopped

—

Yield | 2 servings

To make the bowls, in a medium saucepan, bring the broth to a boil over medium-high heat. Stir in the quinoa, reduce the heat to medium-low, cover, and simmer until the quinoa is tender and the broth has been absorbed, 15 to 20 minutes.

While the quinoa is cooking, combine the chickpeas, tomatoes, olives, cucumber, and onion in a medium bowl. Add the olive oil, lemon juice, oregano, rosemary, dill, salt, and pepper and toss to coat.

To make the sauce, combine all the red pepper sauce ingredients in a food processor and blend on high until smooth, about 1 minute.

Divide the quinoa between 2 bowls. Top each with half of the veggie mixture and a large scoop of roasted red pepper sauce.

ADD IT!

For an additional boost of protein, top each bowl with grilled or roasted chicken breast.

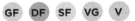
Turmeric "Fried" Rice

Many studies have shown turmeric to be a powerful supplement for brain and body health. It's a potent anti-inflammatory and antioxidant—and makes your food taste good! I love to add turmeric anytime I can, as in this simple side dish, which pairs well with grilled chicken, burgers, or a salad.

1 tablespoon (15 ml) olive oil

1 small yellow onion, diced

1 medium carrot, peeled and finely chopped

3 garlic cloves, minced

1 teaspoon fresh grated ginger

1 teaspoon ground turmeric

½ teaspoon paprika

½ teaspoon salt

¼ teaspoon black pepper

3 cups (585 g) long-grain white or brown rice, rinsed

1 cup (237 ml) well-shaken canned full-fat coconut milk

3 cups (709 ml) vegetable broth

2 cups (260 g) frozen peas

Chopped fresh parsley, for garnish

—

Yield | 12 servings

Heat the olive oil in a large saucepan over medium-high heat. Add the onion and cook, stirring occasionally, until soft and translucent, 2 to 3 minutes. Add the carrot, garlic, ginger, turmeric, paprika, salt, and pepper and stir well to combine. Add the rice and coconut milk and stir, then add the vegetable broth and stir.

Cover, turn the heat to high, and bring to a boil. Turn the heat down to low and simmer for 20 to 25 minutes, until all the liquid is absorbed and the rice is tender. Fluff the rice, then add the peas and mix well. Allow to sit for 5 to 10 minutes until the peas are warmed. Garnish with fresh parsley.

Creamy Penne Arrabbiata

Skip the cream and use cashews to create a dairy-like texture to this pasta sauce. The cashews also help cut the heat from the spicy arrabbiata sauce. It's the perfect combo!

8 ounces (227 g) gluten-free penne (chickpea or brown rice pasta)

1 (24-ounce/680 g) can no-sugar-added arrabbiata pasta sauce

1 cup (145 g) raw, unsalted cashews

½ cup (118 ml) water

1¼ teaspoons sea salt, divided

2 tablespoons (30 ml) olive oil

1 pound (454 g) ground turkey

1 teaspoon garlic powder

Chopped fresh basil and crushed red pepper, for topping

—

Yield | 4 servings

Cook the pasta according to the package directions until al dente. Drain.

While the pasta is cooking, combine the arrabbiata pasta sauce, cashews, water, and ¼ teaspoon of the salt in a food processor or blender. Blend on high for at least 3 minutes, until the cashews are completely broken up and the sauce turns a lighter color. The sauce should be mostly smooth.

In another large saucepan, heat the olive oil over medium heat. Add the ground turkey, sprinkle with the garlic powder and remaining 1 teaspoon salt, and cook, stirring to break up the meat, until cooked through and no longer pink, 3 to 5 minutes.

Turn the heat to low and add the drained pasta and the sauce mixture. Stir to coat and mix the pasta. Top with chopped basil and crushed red pepper.

ADD IT!

You can swap out ground beef or chicken for the ground turkey. Whatever you have on hand works well in this recipe.

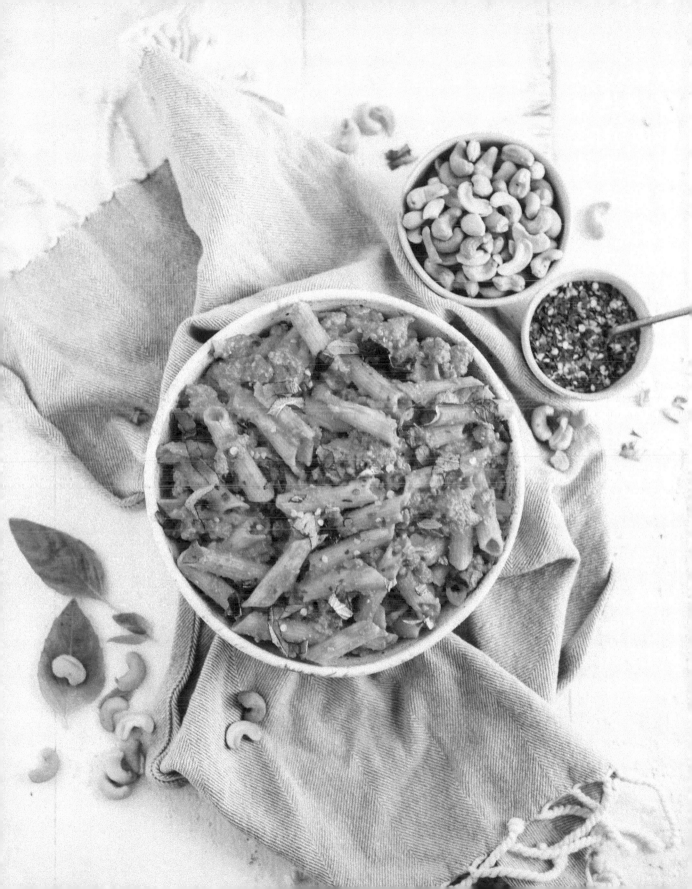

Sausage and Sage Pumpkin Pasta Bake

When the aromas of this meal fill your kitchen, it will immediately take you to a crisp fall day. With cinnamon and a hint of nutmeg, this pasta sauce will warm you up and pleasantly surprise you with the creamy texture the pumpkin gives it.

For the pasta bake:

Nonstick cooking spray

12 ounces (340 g) gluten-free ziti (brown rice or chickpea pasta)

1 tablespoon (14 g) coconut oil

1 pound (454 g) no-sugar-added Italian or traditional sausage, casings removed

1 yellow onion, thinly sliced

2 garlic cloves, minced

4 fresh sage leaves, chopped

1 teaspoon salt

½ teaspoon black pepper

½ teaspoon ground cinnamon

¼ teaspoon ground nutmeg

3 cups (201 g) chopped kale

2 cups (473 ml) chicken broth

½ cup (115 ml) well-shaken canned full-fat coconut milk

1 (15-ounce/425 g) can pumpkin puree

Chopped fresh parsley, for garnish

For the fried sage (optional):

¼ cup (55 g) coconut oil

7 or 8 fresh sage leaves

—

Yield | 8 servings

To make the pasta bake, preheat the oven to 350°F (180°C). Grease a 9 × 13-inch (23 × 33 cm) casserole dish with nonstick cooking spray.

Cook the ziti according to the package directions until al dente. Drain and rinse, then drain again.

While the pasta is cooking, melt the coconut oil in a large skillet over medium-high heat. Add the sausage and cook, breaking it up into small bits, until browned and no pink remains, 2 to 3 minutes. Transfer the sausage to paper towels to drain.

Add the onion to the same skillet and reduce the heat to medium-low. Cook until the onion is caramelized and deep golden brown, about 15 minutes. Add the garlic and sage and cook for 1 to 2 minutes, until fragrant. Add the salt, pepper, cinnamon, and nutmeg and stir well to combine. Add the chopped kale and cook until soft and wilted, about 3 minutes.

Add the chicken broth and coconut milk and mix well, then add the pumpkin puree and stir to combine. Stir in the sausage.

Transfer the cooked pasta to the prepared casserole dish, add the sausage-pumpkin sauce, and stir to completely coat the pasta in sauce. Bake for 25 to 30 minutes, until warmed all the way through and bubbling.

If you want to garnish with fried sage, melt the coconut oil in a skillet over medium-high heat. Add the sage leaves and fry just until crisp, 5 to 10 seconds. Transfer to paper towels to drain, then top the pasta bake with the fried sage and fresh parsley.

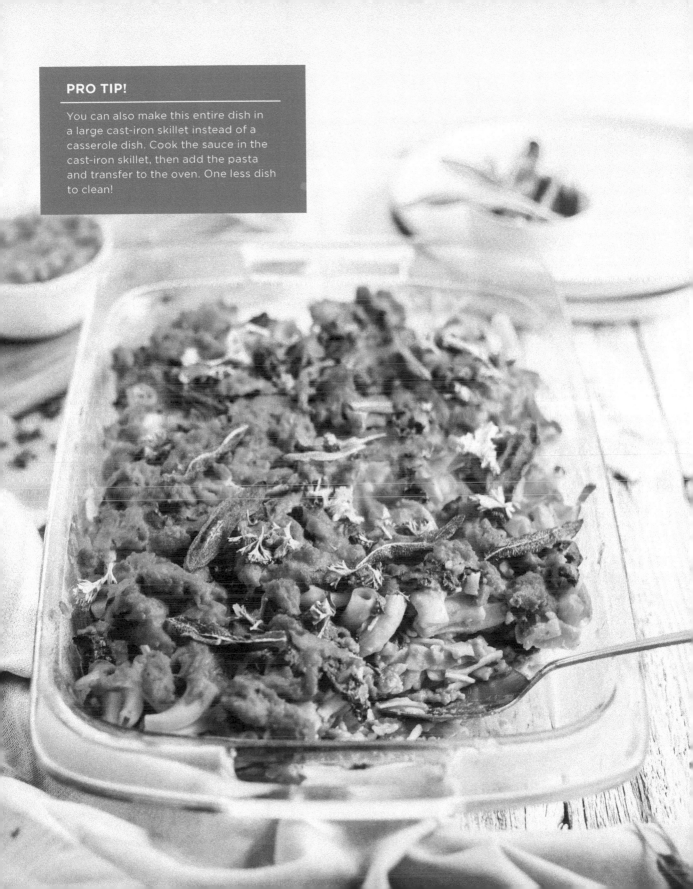

PRO TIP!

You can also make this entire dish in a large cast-iron skillet instead of a casserole dish. Cook the sauce in the cast-iron skillet, then add the pasta and transfer to the oven. One less dish to clean!

Chicken Pad Thai

Pad Thai literally translates to "Thai stir-fry." In the late 1930s, the leader of Thailand wanted to help set the country apart and form a new identity, so he held a competition to create a new national dish. This popular dish was the winner. Its sweet, spicy, salty, and acidic flavors will burst in your mouth!

For the sauce:

¼ cup (63 g) coconut aminos

3 tablespoons (60 g) pure maple syrup

2 tablespoons (30 ml) rice vinegar

2 tablespoons (32 g) peanut butter

Juice of ½ lime

2 teaspoons fish sauce

For the pad Thai:

10 ounces (283 g) Thai rice noodles

2 tablespoons (30 ml) olive oil or avocado oil

1 pound (454 g) boneless, skinless chicken breasts, pounded to 1 inch (2.5 cm) thickness and thinly sliced

1 red bell pepper, seeded and thinly sliced

1 cup (130 g) thinly sliced carrots

2 garlic cloves, minced

5 scallions, thinly sliced on the bias

1 cup (50 g) bean sprouts

3 large eggs

½ cup (75 g) roughly chopped unsalted peanuts or cashews

⅓ cup (20 g) roughly chopped fresh cilantro

Crushed red pepper and sesame seeds, for topping (optional)

—

Yield | 4 servings

To make the sauce, in a small bowl, whisk together all the sauce ingredients; set aside.

To make the pad Thai, cook the rice noodles according to the package directions, then drain, rinse, drain again, and set aside.

Heat the oil in a wok or deep sauté pan over medium-high heat. Add the chicken strips and sauté until cooked through, 5 to 6 minutes. Transfer the chicken to a plate.

Add the bell pepper, carrots, and garlic to the pan and cook for 2 to 3 minutes. Add the scallions and bean sprouts and cook for 1 minute, or until just softened.

Push the veggies to the edges of the pan so there's an empty space in the center of the pan. Crack the eggs into the center and use a silicone spatula to scramble and cook the eggs until just cooked through.

Mix the scrambled eggs and veggies together, then add the chicken, cooked noodles, and sauce. Stir until the noodles are coated and the veggies are thoroughly incorporated. Top with the chopped peanuts and cilantro, then garnish with crushed red pepper and sesame seeds, if desired.

ADD IT!

Feel free to swap out the chicken for shrimp if you're in the mood for seafood. Or leave out the chicken altogether for a vegetarian dish that's still filled with protein, thanks to the eggs.

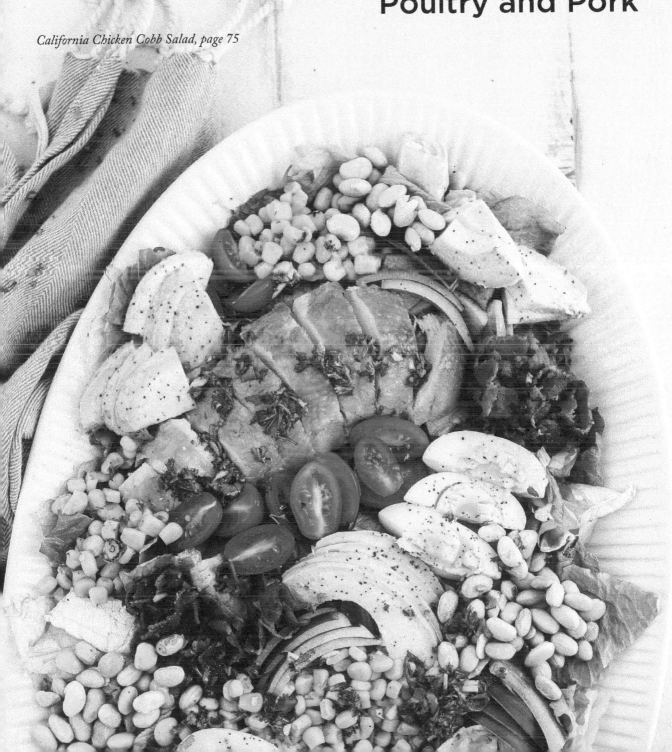

CHAPTER FIVE

Poultry and Pork

California Chicken Cobb Salad, page 75

Sheet Pan Sausage and Veggies

In our house, sheet pan meals make a weekly appearance, and I hope this one becomes a staple in your home. An assortment of veggies and sausage is covered in spices and then roasted to golden brown. Prep ahead of time by chopping all the veggies, then just dump them on the pan when you're ready to roast.

2 teaspoons smoked paprika

1 teaspoon garlic powder

1 teaspoon chili powder

½ teaspoon salt

¼ teaspoon black pepper

13 ounces (369 g) precooked no-sugar-added chicken sausage, sliced diagonally

1 large sweet potato, cut into 2-inch (5 cm) cubes

3½ cups (250 g) small broccoli florets

½ red onion, cut into thick slices

1 red bell pepper, seeded and cut into bite-size pieces

4 garlic cloves, minced

6 tablespoons (90 ml) olive oil

Cooked quinoa or rice, for serving (optional)

Chopped fresh cilantro or parsley, for garnish

—
Yield | 4 servings

Preheat the oven to 400°F (200°C). Line a rimmed baking sheet with aluminum foil or a silicone baking mat.

In a small bowl, combine the smoked paprika, garlic powder, chili powder, salt, and pepper.

Combine the sausage, sweet potato, broccoli, onion, bell pepper, and garlic on the prepared baking sheet. Drizzle the sausage and veggies with the olive oil, sprinkle with the spice mix, and toss to coat well, then spread out in a single layer. Bake for 30 to 40 minutes, stirring every 10 minutes, until browned.

Serve the sausage and veggies over quinoa or rice, if desired, and garnish with cilantro or parsley.

Slow Cooker Chicken Tortilla Soup

Chicken breast cooked low and slow in the slow cooker is one of my favorite ways to eat it. This chicken cooks with broth infused with Mexican spices, and it's so tender it almost falls apart with one fork. We love to make a double batch to take to friends who are busy or maybe just had a baby. If not, we store it in the freezer to thaw on a busy night.

1 (15-ounce/432 g) can black beans, rinsed and drained

1 (14.5-ounce/425 g) can fire-roasted tomatoes

1½ cups (195 g) frozen corn

2 bell peppers (any color), seeded and chopped

3 garlic cloves, minced

1 tablespoon (15 ml) lime juice, plus more for serving

2 cups (473 ml) chicken broth

¼ cup (16 g) chopped fresh cilantro, plus more for serving

1 tablespoon (8 g) chili powder

2 teaspoons ground cumin

2 teaspoons paprika

1 teaspoon salt

½ teaspoon black pepper

1½ pounds (680 g) boneless, skinless chicken breasts

Diced avocado, for serving

—
Yield | 6 servings

Combine all the ingredients, except for the chicken and avocado, in a slow cooker and stir well. Add the chicken breasts, completely submerging them in the soup. Cover and cook on low for 6 to 8 hours, until the chicken reaches an internal temperature of 165°F (74°C).

Transfer the chicken to a cutting board. Shred the meat with two forks. Return the shredded chicken to the soup and stir well. Serve topped with diced avocado, lime juice, and cilantro.

ADD IT!

For a crunchy topping, cut a few corn tortillas into small strips and fry in coconut oil over medium-high heat for a few minutes.

Buffalo Chicken Stuffed Sweet Potatoes

This may seem like an unlikely combo, but it's one you won't soon forget! If you come to our house on a Sunday afternoon, you are almost guaranteed to be welcomed by the smell of Buffalo chicken dip warming in the slow cooker. The key to this recipe is a well-cooked sweet potato. Top with a heaping scoop of Buffalo chicken dip, some homemade ranch, and chopped parsley.

For the Buffalo chicken dip:

1 (2-pound/907 g) rotisserie chicken

1 cup (225 g) paleo mayonnaise

1 cup (230 g) canned coconut cream

1 teaspoon garlic powder

1 teaspoon dried dill

For the sweet potatoes:

6 medium sweet potatoes, well scrubbed

2 tablespoons (28 g) coconut oil, atroom temperature

1 teaspoon sea salt

Dairy-free ranch dressing, for serving

Chopped fresh parsley, for garnish

—

Yield | 6 potatoes

To make the Buffalo chicken dip, remove the skin and bones from the chicken and discard. Shred the meat into bite-size pieces. Put the chicken in a slow cooker, add the mayo, coconut cream, garlic powder, and dill and mix well. Cover and cook on high for 3 to 4 hours, stirring two or three times.

An hour before the slow cooker is done, preheat the oven to 425°F (220°C). Line a rimmed baking sheet with aluminum foil or parchment paper.

To make the sweet potatoes, coat the sweet potatoes with the coconut oil and sprinkle with the salt. Poke each potato with a fork a few times to create steam holes, then place on the prepared baking sheet. Bake for 45 to 60 minutes, until fork-tender. Let them cool for 5 to 10 minutes.

Cut each sweet potato in half lengthwise and add a heaping scoop of the Buffalo chicken dip. Top with ranch and chopped parsley.

ADD IT!

To add some green to your plate, serve the stuffed sweet potatoes with a side of roasted broccoli. Cut a head of broccoli into florets and toss with 1 tablespoon (15 ml) olive oil and a pinch of salt. Add the broccoli to the baking sheet with the sweet potatoes for the last 30 minutes of roasting.

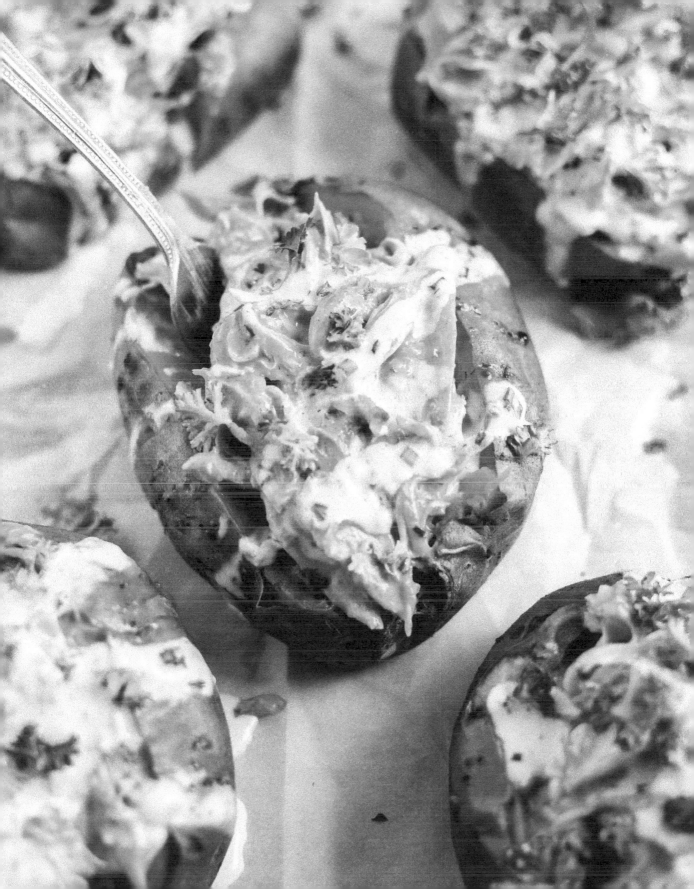

Chicken Parmesan Spaghetti Squash Casserole

It's no secret that spaghetti squash is a low-carb alternative to pasta. Here we bake the spaghetti squash with all your favorite chicken parm ingredients, featuring crispy gluten-free breaded chicken topped with fresh basil.

For the casserole:

1 large spaghetti squash

4 tablespoons (59 ml) olive oil, divided

1 teaspoon salt, divided

¼ teaspoon black pepper

2 garlic cloves, minced

½ medium yellow onion, diced

2 cups (500 g) sugar-free marinara sauce

½ teaspoon crushed red pepper

Chopped fresh basil, for garnish

For the chicken:

1 pound (454 g) boneless, skinless chicken breasts

2 large eggs

1 cup (112 g) almond flour

⅓ cup (43 g) tapioca flour

⅓ teaspoon Italian seasoning

1 teaspoon salt

¼ teaspoon black pepper

¼ cup (55 g) coconut oil

—
Yield | 6 servings

Preheat the oven to 400°F (200°C). Line a rimmed baking sheet with aluminum foil.

To make the casserole, cut the spaghetti squash in half lengthwise, then scoop out and discard the seeds. Drizzle the cut sides of the squash with 2 tablespoons (30 ml) of the olive oil. Season with ½ teaspoon of the salt and the pepper. Place the squash halves, cut-sides down, on the prepared baking sheet and bake for 40 minutes, or until fork tender.

Meanwhile, in a large skillet, heat the remaining 2 tablespoons (30 ml) olive oil over medium heat. Add the garlic and onion and cook until translucent, about 5 minutes. Transfer to a plate and reserve the skillet.

To make the chicken, pound the chicken breasts to about ¼ inch (6 mm) thickness or cut in half horizontally into 2 thin cutlets. Beat the eggs in a medium bowl. In another medium bowl, whisk together the almond flour, tapioca flour, Italian seasoning, salt, and pepper. Pat the chicken dry, then add one piece to the eggs and cover completely. Let the excess drip off, then transfer to the flour mixture and dredge to coat completely. Set aside on a plate and repeat with the remaining chicken breasts.

Melt the coconut oil in the same skillet over medium-high heat. Working in batches as necessary, add the chicken and cook until brown on each side, about 3 minutes on each side. Add more oil as needed to cook all the chicken. When all the chicken is cooked, cut into bite-size pieces.

When the spaghetti squash is done, turn the oven down to 375°F (190°C). Flip the spaghetti squash over and gently run a fork through to separate the spaghetti strands. Transfer the spaghetti squash to a 9 × 13-inch (23 × 33 cm) baking pan. Add 1 cup (250 g) of the marinara, the remaining ½ teaspoon salt, and the crushed red pepper and mix well. Spread the spaghetti squash out to cover the entire pan. Top the spaghetti squash with the remaining 1 cup (250 g) marinara, then arrange the chicken on top. Bake for 30 minutes, until heated through. Top with fresh basil and serve.

PRO TIP!

Save the spaghetti squash seeds to roast for a healthy snack! Toss with olive oil, salt, and pepper and roast at 350°F (180°C) for 15 to 20 minutes.

Caramelized Onion, Kale, and Sausage Stuffed Acorn Squash

There's nothing better than caramelized onions! The natural sugars come out and coat the onions in a dark amber color that translates to a sweet and savory taste that adds depth to any dish. It takes time to cook them down, but it's so worth it!

3 medium acorn squash

2 tablespoons (28 g) coconut oil

1 medium yellow onion

3 garlic cloves, minced

1 pound (454 g) no-sugar-added pork or chicken sausage, casings removed

1 large apple, cored and chopped

4 cups (520 g) roughly chopped kale

1 tablespoon (4 g) finely chopped fresh rosemary

1 tablespoon (4 g) finely chopped fresh sage

2 teaspoons finely chopped fresh thyme

½ teaspoon salt

¼ teaspoon black pepper

—
Yield | 6 stuffed squash

Preheat the oven to 400°F (200°C). Line a rimmed baking sheet with parchment paper or aluminum foil.

Cut the acorn squash in half lengthwise and scoop out the seeds and strings and discard. Place the 6 halves, cut-sides down, on the prepared baking sheet. Roast for 25 to 35 minutes, until the squash is fork-tender.

While the squash is roasting, melt the coconut oil in a large skillet over medium-low heat. Add the onion and cook, stirring frequently, until the onions are very soft and turn amber, 15 to 20 minutes. When the onions are caramelized, add the garlic and cook for 1 to 2 more minutes.

Turn the heat up to medium, add the sausage, and cook, breaking up the meat, until no pink remains, 6 to 8 minutes. Add the apple, kale, rosemary, sage, thyme, salt, and pepper and cook just until the kale wilts.

When the squash is done, remove from the oven and turn the oven to broil. Flip the squash over. Divide the filling evenly among the 6 halves. Broil for 3 to 5 minutes, until the tops get browned and crispy. Let cool slightly before serving.

PRO TIP!

If you can't find sugar-free sausage, you can make your own. In a medium bowl, combine 1 pound (454 g) ground pork with 1 teaspoon fennel seeds, 1 teaspoon dried sage, 1 teaspoon garlic powder, ½ teaspoon onion powder, 1 teaspoon salt, and ½ teaspoon black pepper. Mix well with your hands, then brown as directed.

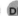

The Best Chicken Soup

Feeling under the weather or just want to cozy up on the couch with a hot cup of soup? This soul-warming chicken soup is packed with immune-boosting ingredients like ginger and turmeric that will fight inflammation and pack a punch of flavor.

1 tablespoon (15 ml) olive oil

6 garlic cloves, minced

1 medium yellow onion, diced

3 large carrots, peeled and thinly sliced into rounds

3 celery stalks, roughly chopped

1 tablespoon (8 g) grated fresh ginger

1 teaspoon ground turmeric

1 teaspoon sea salt

¼ teaspoon black pepper

1 tablespoon (4 g) chopped fresh rosemary

2 teaspoons chopped fresh thyme

6 cups (1420 ml) bone broth or organic chicken broth

1 pound (454 g) boneless, skinless chicken breasts

1 cup (195 g) brown rice

1 cup (130 g) frozen peas

—
Yield | 6 servings

Heat the olive oil in a large Dutch oven or stockpot over medium-high heat. Add the garlic, onion, carrots, and celery and cook, stirring occasionally, for 2 to 3 minutes, until the onion becomes translucent.

Add the ginger, turmeric, salt, and pepper and cook for another 1 to 2 minutes. Add the rosemary, thyme, and broth. Stir briefly to mix, then add the chicken and rice to the pot. Stir to make sure the chicken is completely submerged.

Turn the heat up to high and allow the soup to come to a boil, then reduce the heat to medium-low and simmer for 15 to 20 minutes, until the chicken reaches an internal temperature of 165°F (74°C) and the rice is tender.

Using a slotted spoon, transfer the chicken to a cutting board. Shred the meat with two forks and return it to the soup. Add the frozen peas and stir well to combine.

Store leftovers in an airtight container in the refrigerator for up to 1 week or in the freezer for up to 5 months.

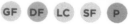

BBQ Chicken Zucchini Boats

The zucchini craze is still going strong, and we've jumped on board this trend by using hollowed-out zucchini instead of a bun or bread to hold BBQ chicken. It's a great way to add greens to your day if you aren't feeling a salad. Zucchini is a great source of vitamins A and C, potassium, and fiber.

For the zucchini boats:

Nonstick cooking spray

4 medium zucchini, cut in half lengthwise

1 tablespoon (15 ml) olive oil

½ red onion, diced

2 garlic cloves, minced

1 pound (454 g) shredded cooked chicken breast (or rotisserie chicken)

Chopped red onion, avocado, scallions, cilantro, and/or pineapple, for topping

Dairy-free ranch dressing for topping

For the BBQ sauce:

1 (14.5-ounce/425 g) can tomato sauce

⅓ cup (79 ml) apple cider vinegar

3 tablespoons (60 g) pure maple syrup

1 tablespoon (12 g) spicy brown mustard

1 tablespoon (16 g) tomato paste

1 tablespoon (8 g) smoked paprika

1 teaspoon onion powder

1 teaspoon garlic powder

½ teaspoon salt

—
Yield | 8 zucchini boats

To make the zucchini boats, preheat the oven to 400°F (200°C). Coat a rimmed baking sheet with nonstick cooking spray.

Use a large spoon to hollow out the centers of each zucchini half, leaving about ½ inch (1.25 cm) rim to create boats. Place the zucchini on the prepared baking sheet and coat lightly with nonstick cooking spray.

To make the BBQ sauce, in a small bowl, whisk together all the BBQ sauce ingredients and set aside.

In a medium skillet, heat the olive oil over medium heat. Add the onion and cook, stirring frequently, until softened and translucent, about 3 minutes. Add the garlic and cook for 1 to 2 minutes, until fragrant. Transfer the onion and garlic to a large bowl and add the chicken.

Add most of the prepared BBQ sauce to the bowl, leaving a few tablespoons aside for topping, and mix well to coat the chicken.

Spoon the BBQ chicken mixture evenly into the prepared zucchini boats, then top each with a little of the remaining BBQ sauce. Bake for 20 to 25 minutes, until the zucchini is completely heated through and fork-tender.

Serve with your favorite toppings.

PRO TIP!

There are a few ways you can cook the chicken for this recipe: oven, pressure cooker, or slow cooker. For the oven, bake at 400°F (200°C) for 15 to 20 minutes. For the pressure cooker, cook with 1 cup (237 ml) chicken broth on high for 15 minutes, then use natural release for 5 minutes. For the slow cooker, cook with 1 cup (237 ml) chicken broth on low for 3 hours.

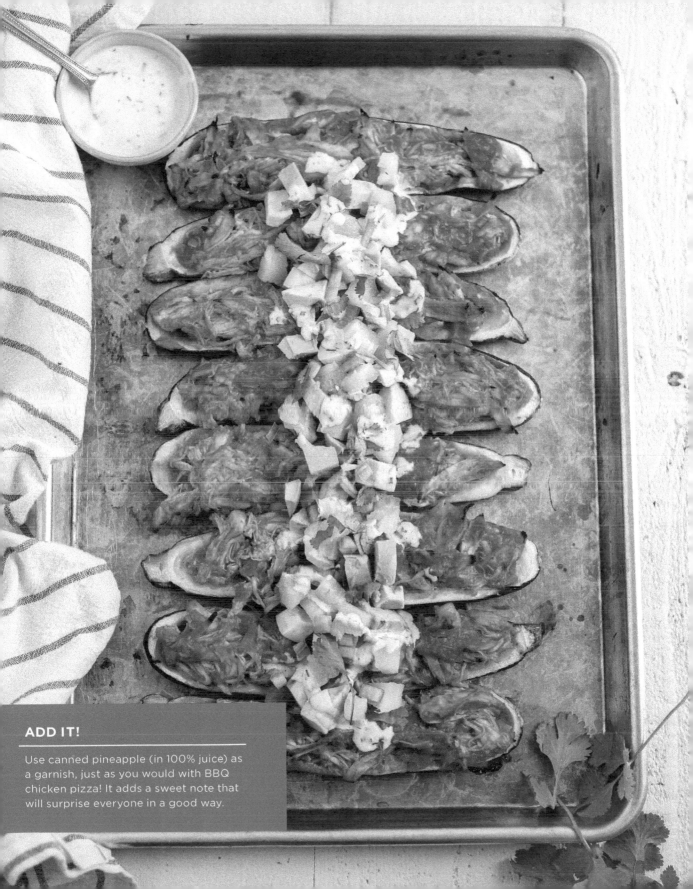

ADD IT!

Use canned pineapple (in 100% juice) as a garnish, just as you would with BBQ chicken pizza! It adds a sweet note that will surprise everyone in a good way.

Everything Bagel Chicken Salad

Is there anything you can't put everything bagel seasoning on? We've loved it on avocado toast and eggs for years, but now we can't get enough of this chicken salad. It takes just minutes to make. Serve on your favorite gluten-free bread or on a bed of lettuce and tomato.

1 (2-pound/907 g) rotisserie chicken

1 cup (150 g) grapes, halved

1 celery stalk, finely chopped

¼ cup (40 g) dicedred onion

2 tablespoons (16 g) everything bagel seasoning

1 cup (225 g) paleo mayonnaise

2 teaspoons Dijon mustard

Juice of ½ lemon

Chopped fresh parsley, for garnish

—
Yield | 6 cups (1.5 kg)

Remove the skin and bones from the chicken and discard. Shred the meat into bite-size pieces and put it in a large bowl. Add the remaining ingredients and stir until the chicken is coated. Serve, topped with parsley.

Dad's Best Turkey Chili

Every year my dad makes a big batch of his famous chili on Christmas Eve and we all watch a Christmas movie together. When I met my husband, I discovered that his family always eats chili on Christmas Day. We decided from then on that we were going to carry on the tradition with our family. Now we have chili on Christmas Eve and Christmas Day. (No such thing as too much of my dad's chili!) This recipe reminds me of home and the holidays and brings back the best memories. I hope you love this recipe so much it helps you start fun traditions in your home.

1 tablespoon (15 ml) olive oil

1 medium yellow onion, chopped

1 red bell pepper, seeded and chopped

1 pound (454 g) ground turkey

1 pound (454 g) no-sugar-added Italian sausage, casings removed

2 (14.5-ounce/425g) cans diced tomatoes, drained

2 (15-ounce/432 g) cans black beans, rinsed and drained

1 (15-ounce/425 g) can sweet corn, drained

1 (15-ounce/425 g) can tomato sauce

2 tablespoons (15 g) smoked paprika

2 teaspoons chili powder

2 teaspoons coconut sugar

1 teaspoon ground cumin

1 teaspoon garlic powder

1 teaspoon onion powder

1 teaspoon salt

½ teaspoon black pepper

Chopped fresh cilantro, scallions, and/or avocado, for topping

—

Yield | 6 servings

Heat the olive oil in a large stockpot over medium heat. Add the onion and bell pepper and cook, stirring occasionally, for about 3 minutes, until soft. Add the ground turkey and Italian sausage and cook, breaking up the meat, until no pink remains, 3 to 5 minutes.

Add the remaining ingredients and mix well to incorporate. Cover and bring to a boil over medium-high heat, then reduce the heat and simmer for 20 minutes. Serve with your favorite toppings.

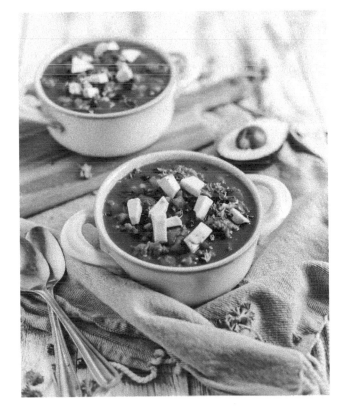

Buffalo Chicken and Broccoli Quinoa Casserole

Chicken and quinoa provide healthy carbs and protein for this recipe, and the healthy fats come from mayo and coconut cream. I've added a little extra broccoli for a boost of vitamin K, folate, and potassium. You can't have too many greens in an anti-inflammatory diet!

1 pound (454 g) boneless, skinless chicken breasts

1½ cups (355 ml) chicken broth

1 cup (173 g) quinoa

3½ cups (249 g) broccoli florets

1 tablespoon (15 ml) lemon juice

1 teaspoon garlic powder

1 teaspoon paprika

1 teaspoon dried dill

1½ teaspoons dried chives

1 teaspoon salt

¼ teaspoon black pepper

½ cup (115 g) paleo mayonnaise

½ cup (115 g) canned coconut cream

⅓ cup (83 g) hot sauce

Chopped scallions, for serving

—
Yield | 8 servings

In a slow cooker, combine the chicken, broth, quinoa, broccoli, lemon juice, garlic powder, paprika, dried dill, dried chives, salt, and pepper. Stir well to combine. Cover and cook on low for 6 hours or on high for 3 hours.

Transfer the chicken breasts to a cutting board. Shred the meat using two forks, then return the meat to the slow cooker. Add the mayo, coconut cream, and hot sauce and mix well to combine. Cover and cook on high for 20 more minutes to heat. Serve topped with scallions.

Slow Cooker Chicken Curry

Spices like turmeric and ginger have long been used in Indian cuisine to help fight inflammation. This dish features tender chunks of chicken swimming in a creamy (dairy-free!) curry sauce. We love to serve it over a bed of rice.

2 teaspoons ground coriander

2 teaspoons ground cumin

1 teaspoon ground turmeric

1 teaspoon sea salt

¼ teaspoon black pepper

1 pound (454 g) boneless, skinless chicken breasts or thighs, cut into 1-inch (2.5 cm) pieces

2 tablespoons (28 g) coconut oil

1 small yellow onion, diced

3 garlic cloves, minced

1 tablespoon (8 g) grated fresh ginger

3 tablespoons (45 g) red curry paste

1 large red bell pepper, seeded and thinly sliced

1 (13.5-ounce/383 g) can full-fat coconut milk

Juice of ½ lime

1 tablespoon (20 g) pure maple syrup

1 tablespoon (8 g) tapioca flour

1 tablespoon (15 ml) water

Cooked basmati rice or cauliflower rice, for serving

Chopped fresh cilantro, for garnish

—

Yield | 6 servings

Combine the coriander, cumin, turmeric, salt, and pepper in a medium bowl. Add the chicken and toss to coat.

Melt the coconut oil in a large skillet over medium-high heat. Add the onion and cook, stirring frequently, until soft and translucent, 3 to 4 minutes. Add the garlic, ginger, and red curry paste and cook for another 1 to 2 minutes. Add the seasoned chicken and cook, stirring frequently, for 4 to 5 minutes, until the chicken is browned on all sides.

Transfer the contents of the skillet to a slow cooker. Add the coconut milk, lime juice, and maple syrup and stir to combine. Cover and cook on low for 5 to 6 hours or on high for 3 hours.

In a small bowl, whisk together the tapioca flour and water. Add the mixture to the slow cooker and stir well. Cover and cook on high for 20 minutes to thicken. Serve over rice, garnished with cilantro.

PRO TIP!

To prep this recipe in advance, cook the onion and brown the chicken in a skillet over medium-high heat, then combine it with all the remaining ingredients in a large resealable plastic bag and refrigerate overnight. In the morning, dump the contents into the slow cooker and cook on low for 8 hours while you're at work. Follow the directions to thicken the sauce.

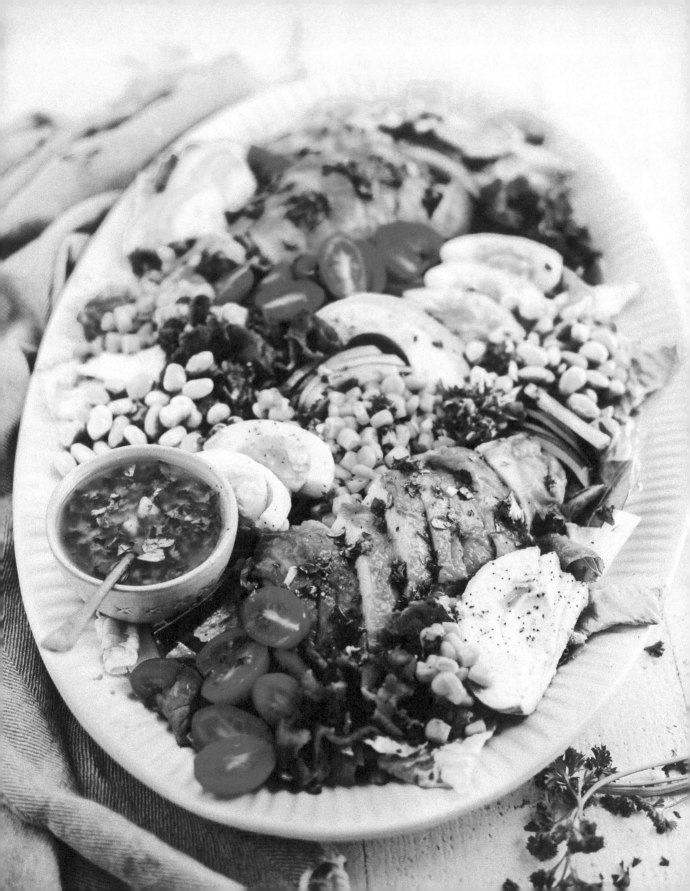

California Chicken Cobb Salad

Just imagine you're sitting on the patio of a coastal restaurant in California enjoying every bite of this fresh, protein-packed salad. I like to make a double batch of this herb vinaigrette—I pour it on everything I can!

For the salad:

8 ounces (226 g) nitrate-free, sugar-free bacon

8 cups (240 g) mixed greens

2 (3-ounce/85 g) boneless, skinless cooked chicken breasts (or rotisserie chicken), sliced

3 hard-boiled eggs, quartered

1 large avocado, peeled, pitted, and sliced

¼ cup (80 g) thinly sliced red onion

½ cup (75 g) edamame, shelled

½ cup (75 g) grape tomatoes, cut in half

1 (15-ounce/425 g) can fire-roasted corn, drained

For the herb vinaigrette:

½ cup (118 g) light olive oil

6 tablespoons (90 ml) red wine vinegar

2 tablespoons (40 g) raw honey

2 teaspoons Dijon mustard

1 garlic clove, minced

2 tablespoons (8 g) chopped fresh parsley

2 tablespoons (8 g) chopped fresh cilantro

½ teaspoon sea salt

¼ teaspoon black pepper

—
Yield | 4 servings

To make the salad, heat a skillet over medium-high heat and add the bacon. Brown until crisp, 2 to 3 minutes on each side, then transfer to paper towels to drain. When it's cool enough to handle, crumble into bite-size pieces.

Put the mixed greens on a large salad plate or in a bowl, then top with the chicken, hard-boiled eggs, avocado, red onion, edamame, tomatoes, corn, and crumbled bacon.

To make the vinaigrette, combine all the herb vinaigrette ingredients in a bowl and whisk well, or combine in a jar with a lid and shake well (or whisk together in a small bowl). Top the salad with the dressing and serve.

ADD IT!

Don't love cilantro? Swap it out for another favorite herb, like basil.

Tuscan Sausage and Cauliflower Soup

Tuscan soup is a classic Italian soup typically made with sausage, potatoes, and a creamy broth. This healthier version is gluten- and dairy-free, and made with cauliflower instead of potatoes. It's a perfect meal for people who are being mindful of their carb intake.

1 tablespoon (15 ml) olive oil

1 pound (454 g) no-sugar-added Italian sausage, casings removed

1 medium white onion, diced

3 garlic cloves, minced

6 cups (1429 ml) reduced-sodium chicken broth or bone broth

3½ cups (462 g) cauliflower florets

1 teaspoon salt

½ teaspoon crushed red pepper

4 cups (268 g) stemmed and chopped kale

1 cup (230 g) canned coconut cream

1 tablespoon (8 g) tapioca flour

—
Yield | 6 servings

Heat the oil in a Dutch oven or stockpot over medium-high heat. Add the sausage and cook, breaking up the meat, until browned and no pink remains, 3 to 5 minutes.

Add the onion and cook for 2 to 3 minutes, until softened, then add the garlic and cook for another 30 seconds. Add the broth, cauliflower, salt, and crushed red pepper and bring to a boil. Boil until the cauliflower is fork-tender, about 10 minutes. Add the kale and coconut cream and stir to combine. Cook until the kale is wilted and tender, about 3 minutes.

Remove ½ cup (118 ml) of the broth to a small bowl and whisk in the tapioca flour to create a slurry. Pour the slurry back into the soup and cook for 3 to 5 minutes, until smooth and thickened.

Turkey-Sage Swedish Meatballs with Creamy Spinach Gravy

Dairy-free, gluten-free meatballs with a thick, creamy gravy make such a comforting and filling meal. This recipe is an anti-inflammatory version of the classic Swedish dish. Dark leafy greens are some of the best ingredients you can eat for fighting inflammation, and spinach is one of the best known of all. Six cups of spinach may seem like a lot, but it wilts down and still gives you all those nutrients like iron, vitamin A, and magnesium.

For the meatballs:

1 pound (454 g) ground turkey

1 large egg

¼ cup (32 g) tapioca flour

2 tablespoons (16 g) coconut flour

3 tablespoons (12 g) chopped fresh sage

1 tablespoon (4 g) chopped fresh thyme

2 teaspoons chopped fresh rosemary

½ teaspoon garlic powder

½ teaspoon onion powder

½ teaspoon fine sea salt

⅛ teaspoon black pepper

1 tablespoon (14 g) coconut oil

For the gravy:

3 tablespoons (42 g) ghee or coconut oil

2¼ cups (591 ml) chicken broth

1 tablespoon (8 g) tapioca flour

2 tablespoons (32 g) coconut aminos

1 teaspoon Dijon mustard

½ teaspoon sea salt

¼ teaspoon black pepper

6 cups (180 g) fresh baby spinach

Mashed potatoes, for serving (optional)

—

Yield | 4 servings

To make the meatballs, in a large bowl, combine all the meatball ingredients, except for the oil, and mix well using a wooden spoon or your clean hands. Scoop out 1 tablespoon (15 g) of the mixture and roll into 1¼- to 1½-inch (3 to 4 cm) meatballs. The mixture will be wet and sticky. You can add a little tapioca flour to your hands to help keep them from sticking. You should get about 20 meatballs.

Melt the coconut oil in a deep sauté pan over medium heat. Working in batches if necessary, fry the meatballs until they are browned on all sides and cooked through (they should reach an internal temperature of 165°F/74°C), about 3 minutes on each side. Transfer the meatballs to a plate and tent with aluminum foil.

To make the gravy, melt the coconut oil in the same pan over medium-low heat. In a large liquid measuring cup, whisk together the broth and tapioca flour until dissolved. Add the mixture to the pan and whisk continuously for 3 to 4 minutes, until the mixture is simmering and starting to thicken. Whisk in the coconut aminos, mustard, salt, and pepper. Add the spinach and stir until soft and wilted.

Return the meatballs to the pan and stir well to combine. Serve the meatballs and gravy over mashed potatoes if desired.

PRO TIP!

Use a cookie scoop to form the meatballs.

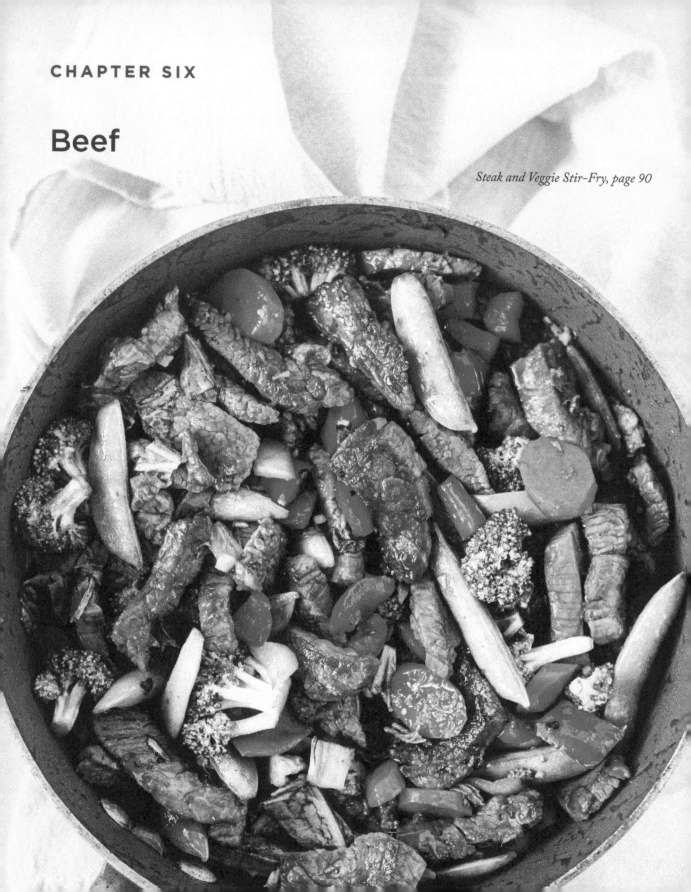

CHAPTER SIX

Beef

Steak and Veggie Stir-Fry, page 90

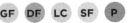

Instant Pot Mongolian Beef

This is one of the most popular recipes on What Molly Made, so I couldn't write a cookbook without sharing it with all of you! It's done in less than 20 minutes and is delicious served over a bed of rice.

½ cup (118 ml) water

⅓ cup (80 ml) coconut aminos

4 garlic cloves, minced

1 teaspoon grated fresh ginger

1½ pounds (680 g) flank steak, thinly sliced against the grain

1 tablespoon (8 g) tapioca flour

¼ cup (85 g) raw honey

2 cups (142 g) chopped broccoli

Cooked quinoa or brown rice, for serving (optional)

Sesame seeds and chopped scallions, for topping

—

Yield | 6 to 8 servings

In a small bowl, whisk together the water, coconut aminos, garlic, and ginger.

Set the pressure cooker to sauté mode. Allow it to heat up, then add the steak (without any oil) and sear quickly on each side for about 20 seconds. Cancel sauté mode and pour the liquid mixture over the browned steak. Lock the lid, press the manual (or pressure cook) button, and adjust the time to 11 minutes.

When the time is up, release the vent all at once using the handle of a wooden spoon to avoid the jet of hot steam. When the pressure has come down, unlock the lid and transfer 2 tablespoons (30 ml) of the cooking liquid to a small bowl. Add the tapioca flour and whisk to dissolve. Pour the mixture into the pressure cooker, add the honey, and stir well. Add the chopped broccoli, set the pressure cooker to sauté mode again, and allow it to boil for 3 to 5 minutes, until the sauce is thickened.

Serve the beef over brown rice or quinoa if you like, and top with sesame seeds and scallions.

PRO TIP!

The muscle fibers run length-wise on a cut of flank steak. Cutting against the grain means you should cut your steak perpendicular to the grain to help shorten the fibers. This makes it more tender and easier to chew.

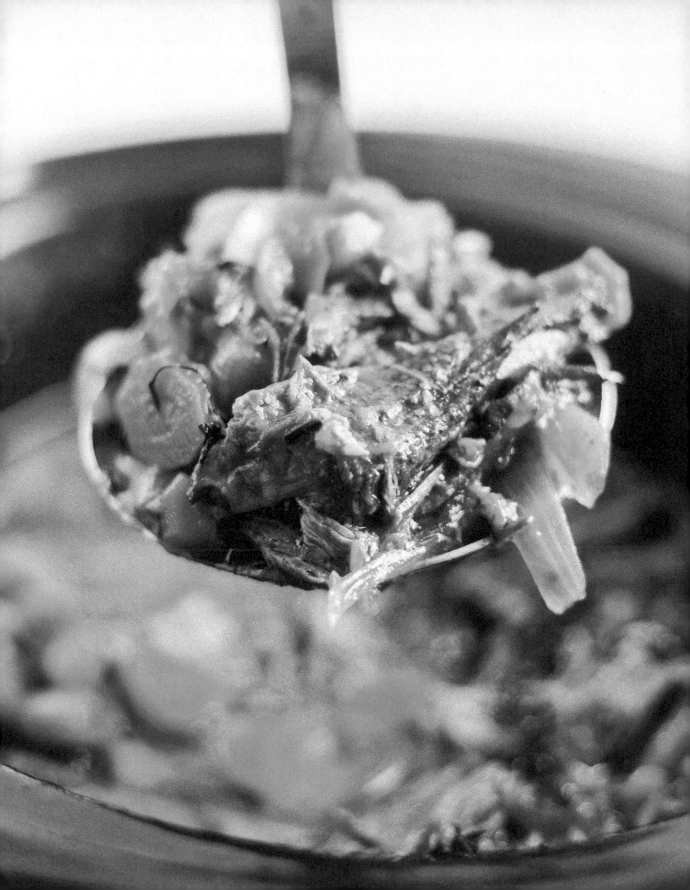

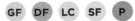

Slow Cooker Pot Roast

The tough tissue in a pot roast makes it great for cooking low and slow in your slow cooker. When you open the lid, the beef just falls apart. This recipe is perfect for a crisp fall night.

Nonstick cooking spray

8 ounces (227 g) cremini mushrooms, sliced

1 medium yellow onion, sliced

4 medium carrots, peeled and sliced

3 celery stalks, cut into 1-inch (2.5 cm) pieces

2 medium sweet potatoes, peeled and cut into 1-inch (2.5 cm) cubes

1 (2½-pound/1134 g) chuck roast

1 teaspoon salt

⅛ teaspoon black pepper

2 tablespoons (30 ml) olive oil or coconut oil

1¼ cups (315 ml) beef broth or bone broth

1 tablespoon (16 g) coconut aminos

1 tablespoon (4 g) chopped fresh thyme

1 tablespoon (4 g) chopped fresh rosemary

—

Yield | 8 servings

Coat a large slow cooker with nonstick cooking spray, then add the mushrooms, onion, carrots, celery, and sweet potatoes.

Season the chuck roast with the salt and pepper. Heat the olive oil in a skillet over medium-high heat. Add the roast and brown for about 30 seconds per side, then transfer to the slow cooker on top of the veggies. Add the broth, coconut aminos, thyme, and rosemary. Cover and cook on low for 10 hours.

Using two forks, shred the beef in the pot and stir to mix it in with the vegetables.

PRO TIP!

If you have a pressure cooker, you can make this in just an hour! Set it to sauté mode and sear the chuck roast on all sides. Add the rest of the ingredients and pressure cook on high for 1 hour. If your chuck roast is smaller or larger than what the recipe calls for, add or subtract 10 minutes from the cook time per pound (454 g) of roast.

Chili Stuffed Sweet Potatoes

Maybe you serve your chili with cornbread, but have you ever had it served over a sweet potato? We think pretty much anything can be stuffed inside a sweet potato, but chili is especially good!

For the sweet potatoes:

4 medium sweet potatoes, well scrubbed

1 tablespoon (14 g) coconut oil, at room temperature

½ teaspoon salt

For the chili:

1 tablespoon (14 g) coconut oil

1 medium yellow onion, diced

1 large bell pepper (any color), seeded and diced

3 garlic cloves, minced

1 pound (454 g) ground beef

1 pound (454 g) no-sugar-added Italian sausage, casings removed, or ground pork

1 (28-ounce/794 g) can diced tomatoes, undrained

1¾ cups (414 ml) beef broth or bone broth

2 tablespoons (32 g) tomato paste

2 tablespoons (16 g) smoked paprika

2 teaspoons chili powder

1 teaspoon ground cumin

1 teaspoon garlic powder

1 teaspoon onion powder

1 teaspoon sea salt

½ teaspoon black pepper

Chopped fresh cilantro, diced red onion, or diced avocado, for topping

—

Yield | 4 servings

Preheat the oven to 425°F (220°C). Line a medium baking pan with a silicone baking mat or aluminum foil.

To make the sweet potatoes, coat the sweet potatoes with the coconut oil and sprinkle with the salt. Poke each potato with a fork a few times to create steam holes, then place on the prepared baking sheet. Bake for 50 to 60 minutes, or until fork-tender.

While the sweet potatoes are baking, prepare the chili. Melt the coconut oil in a medium stockpot over medium-high heat. Add the onion and bell pepper and cook, stirring occasionally, until the onion is soft and translucent, 3 to 5 minutes. Add the garlic and

cook for another 1 to 2 minutes. Add the ground beef and sausage and cook, breaking up the meat, and cook until browned and no pink remains, about 5 minutes. Add the rest of the ingredients and stir well to combine. Cover and bring to a gentle boil over medium heat, then reduce the heat to a simmer and cook, covered, for 30 minutes, stirring occasionally.

When the potatoes are done, allow them to cool slightly so they're cool enough to handle. Cut them in half lengthwise and open them up. Ladle a large scoop of chili inside each sweet potato. Serve with your favorite toppings.

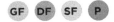

Short Ribs with Potatoes and Veggies

The fall-off-the-bone ribs you get at your favorite restaurant can be made right at home with healthy ingredients. This entire meal is gluten- and dairy-free, plus you get all the essential amino acids from the beef and nutrients from the carrots, celery, tomatoes, and potatoes. Feel good about serving this comfort food to your family!

2 teaspoons coconut oil

6 (10-ounce/283 g) bone-in beef short ribs

1 **teaspoon** salt

1 teaspoon black pepper

4 garlic cloves, minced

1 large yellow onion, diced

2 celery stalks, sliced

2 carrots, peeled and chopped

3 cups (710 ml) beef broth

1 cup (237 ml) water

3 tablespoons (48 g) tomato paste

1 tablespoon (16 g) coconut aminos

2 bay leaves

2 fresh thyme sprigs

1 fresh rosemary sprig

1 pound (454 g) small red potatoes

—
Yield | 6 servings

Preheat the oven to 325°F (170°C).

Melt the coconut oil in a large Dutch oven over medium-high heat. Season both sides of the ribs with the salt and pepper. Sear the ribs for 2 to 3 minutes per side to create a deep crust. Transfer the ribs to a cutting board. Add the garlic, onion, celery, and carrots to the pan and cook, stirring frequently, for 8 to 10 minutes, until the veggies turn a deep caramel color.

Add the broth, water, tomato paste, and coconut aminos and stir, scraping up any brown bits from the bottom of the pan. Add the bay leaves, thyme, and rosemary, then add the seared beef. The braising liquid should come about halfway up

the sides of the ribs. Bring the liquid to a simmer, then cover and transfer to the oven for 1 hour 45 minutes.

Remove from the oven, add the potatoes, cover, and return to the oven for 45 more minutes to finish cooking. The ribs should be tender and easily fall apart.

Carefully transfer the ribs and potatoes to a platter, leaving just the braising liquid in the pot. Tent the platter with aluminum foil to keep warm. Remove the bay leaves and herb sprigs from the pot and set the pot over medium-low heat. Cook for 5 to 10 minutes to reduce and thicken the braising liquid. Serve the beef and potatoes and spoon the braising liquid on top.

Flank Steak with Kale Chimichurri

Fresh herbs make every meal better! Chimichurri is a South American condiment often served with grilled meat. The finely chopped herbs have an aromatic flavor, while the lemon and vinegar give the sauce a tangy punch. I added fresh kale to this recipe because it's full of vitamin K, an anti-inflammatory powerhouse.

For the kale chimichurri:

½ cup (34 g) stemmed and roughly chopped kale

1 cup (60 g) tightly packed fresh cilantro

½ cup (30 g) tightly packed fresh parsley

½ cup (80 g) roughly chopped red onion

3 garlic cloves, peeled

3 tablespoons (45 ml) red wine vinegar

2 tablespoons (30 ml) lemon juice

½ teaspoon salt

¼ teaspoon black pepper

½ cup (118 ml) extra-virgin olive oil

For the steak:

1½ pounds (680 g) flank steak

1 teaspoon salt

½ teaspoon black pepper

—

Yield | 6 servings

To make the kale chimichurri, combine all the ingredients, except the olive oil, in a food processor. Pulse for 2 to 3 minutes, until all the ingredients are finely chopped. With the machine running, slowly add the olive oil through the feed tube and blend until it's completely incorporated.

To make the steak, pat the steak dry, then season with the salt and pepper. Put the steak in a resealable plastic bag, add 3 tablespoons (48 g) of the chimichurri, and press the bag to coat the steak all over with the chimichurri. Seal the bag and allow the steak to marinate at room temperature for 15 minutes or in the refrigerator up to overnight.

(If marinating for longer than 1 hour, also refrigerate the rest of the chimichurri in an airtight container.)

Turn on the oven broiler. Line a rimmed baking sheet with aluminum foil.

Transfer the marinated steak to the prepared baking sheet and broil for 5 to 7 minutes. When the time is up and the steak is starting to turn brown, flip the steak and broil the other side for an additional 5 to 7 minutes, until it reaches an internal temperature of 140°F to 145°F (60°C to 63°C). Transfer the steak to a cutting board to rest for 10 to 15 minutes, then slice thinly against the grain. Serve with the rest of the chimichurri.

PRO TIP!

Cook your steak between 140°F and 145°F (60°C and 63°C) for medium-rare steak. This allows for carryover cooking while the steak is resting. Cook your steak to 150°F (65°C) for medium-well.

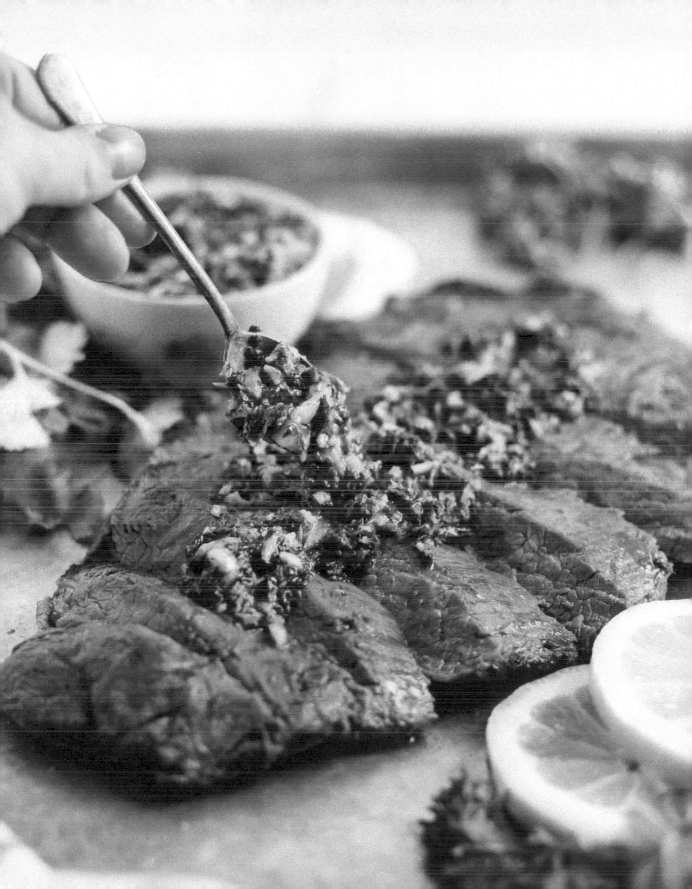

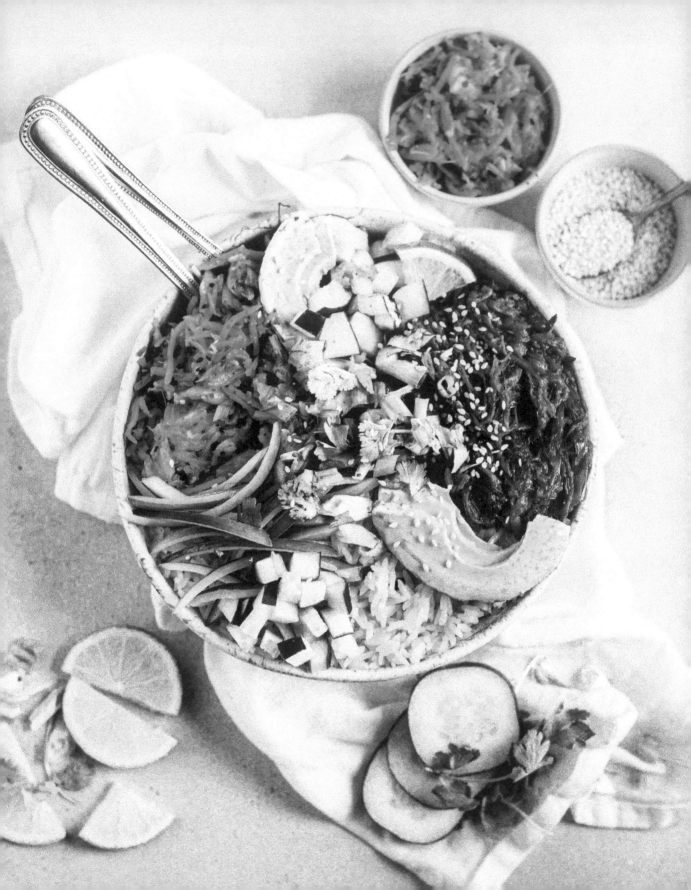

Slow Cooker Korean Barbacoa Bowls

I bet this is some of the most flavorful beef you'll have in a long time! The longer and slower you cook this cut of beef, the more the fibrous tissue and fat melt, which makes it rich and flavorful. Pair it with probiotic-rich kimchi for a full anti-inflammatory meal.

For the beef:

2 tablespoons (28 g) coconut oil

1 (2-pound/907 g) chuck roast

1 teaspoon salt

½ teaspoon black pepper

1 medium yellow onion, thinly sliced

3 garlic cloves, minced

1 tablespoon (8 g) grated fresh ginger

¼ cup (59 ml) beef broth

½ cup (125 g) coconut aminos

1 tablespoon (20 g) pure maple syrup

1 teaspoon toasted sesame oil (optional)

2 tablespoons (16 g) tapioca flour

For the sriracha mayo:

¼ cup (60 g) paleo mayonnaise

1 tablespoon (15 g) sriracha

2 teaspoons lime juice

For the bowls:

4 cups (800 g) cooked white or brown rice

1 cup (160 g) sliced red onion

½ cucumber, diced

2 avocados, peeled, pitted, and sliced

1 cup (90 g) kimchi

Sesame seeds, chopped fresh cilantro, and chopped scallions, for garnish

—

Yield | 4 servings

To make the beef, melt the coconut oil in a large skillet over high heat. Season both sides of the chuck roast with the salt and pepper. Sear the roast for 3 to 4 minutes per side to create a crust that seals in the juices. Transfer the beef to a slow cooker. Add the onion, garlic, ginger, broth, coconut aminos, maple syrup, and sesame oil (if using). Cover and cook on low for 10 hours.

Using two forks, shred the beef in the pot. Transfer 2 tablespoons (30 ml) of the liquid to a small bowl. Add the tapioca flour and whisk to dissolve, then pour the mixture into the slow cooker. Cover and cook on high for 20 minutes to thicken.

Meanwhile, to make the sriracha mayo, in a small bowl, whisk together the mayo, sriracha, and lime juice. Cover and refrigerate until ready to use.

To assemble the bowl, fill each bowl with rice and top with shredded beef, red onion, cucumber, avocado, and kimchi. Garnish with sesame seeds, cilantro, and scallions. Drizzle with the sriracha mayo.

Veggie-Packed Shepherd's Pie

Traditional shepherd's pie uses lamb, but this version with beef is widely known as well. It's full of healthy veggies and covered with a creamy mashed potato topping that turns crispy golden brown in the oven.

For the shepherd's pie:

2 tablespoons (28 g) coconut oil

1 small yellow onion, chopped

2 garlic cloves, minced

2 celery stalks, chopped

2 carrots, peeled and chopped

8 ounces (227 g) cremini mushrooms, sliced

1 pound (454 g) ground beef

1 teaspoon salt

¼ teaspoon black pepper

1 cup (130 g) frozen peas

1 (14.5-ounce/432 g) can fire-roasted diced tomatoes, undrained

1½ cups (355 ml) beef broth

2 tablespoons (32 g) tomato paste

2 tablespoons (32 g) coconut aminos

2 tablespoons (16 g) tapioca flour

1 fresh rosemary sprig

3 fresh thyme sprigs

2 bay leaves

For the potatoes:

2 pounds (907 g) Yukon gold potatoes (about 6 medium potatoes), peeled and cut into chunks

½ cup (115 g) canned coconut cream

¼ cup (59 g) coconut oil

¼ cup (59 ml) unsweetened nondairy milk

1 teaspoon sea salt

¼ teaspoon black pepper

1 tablespoon (15 ml) olive oil, for drizzling (optional)

—

Yield | 6 to 8 servings

Preheat the oven to 350°F (180°C).

To make the shepherd's pie, melt the coconut oil in a large cast-iron skillet over medium heat. Add the onion and cook, stirring frequently, for 2 to 3 minutes, until soft and translucent. Add the garlic and cook for an additional 1 to 2 minutes. Add the celery, carrots, and mushrooms and cook for 3 to 4 minutes, until the vegetables are softened and the mushrooms have shrunk down.

Turn the heat up to medium-high and add the ground beef, salt, and pepper. Cook, breaking up the meat, until browned and no longer pink, 3 to 5 minutes. Drain any excess fat from the pan if needed, then turn the heat back down to medium. Add the frozen peas, diced tomatoes, broth, tomato paste, and coconut aminos and stir well to combine.

Transfer 2 to 3 tablespoons (30 to 45 ml) of the liquid to a small bowl. Add the tapioca flour and whisk to dissolve. Pour the mixture into the pot and stir well to combine. Add the rosemary, thyme, and bay leaves, then turn the heat to medium-low and allow to simmer and thicken for about 5 minutes. Remove the herbs, then allow to cool at room temperature while you make the potatoes. Cooling the mixture helps create a definitive line between the filling and the potatoes.

To make the potatoes, put the potatoes in a medium stockpot and pour in enough water to cover by about 1 inch (2.5 cm). Bring to a boil over medium-high heat and boil for 5 to 8 minutes, until the potatoes are fork-tender. Drain the potatoes and return them to the pot. Add the coconut cream, coconut oil, milk, salt, and pepper. Use a handheld mixer, the back of a fork, or a potato masher to mix everything together until smooth.

Spread the mashed potatoes evenly over the top of the veggie mixture, getting it as close as you can to the edges of the pan. Drizzle with olive oil if desired and bake for 15 to 20 minutes. If you like, turn the oven to broil for 3 to 5 minutes at the end to brown the top of the potatoes.

Steak and Veggie Stir-Fry

Stir-fries are great weeknight dinners because they require just one pan and let you use up whatever you have in the fridge. This recipe calls for broccoli, carrots, and snap peas, but so many veggies marry well with these Asian flavors that you can use whatever you have on hand. The more veggies, the better for an anti-inflammatory diet.

½ cup (118 ml) beef broth

⅓ cup (83 g) coconut aminos

2 tablespoons (40 g) pure maple syrup

1 teaspoon grated fresh ginger

1 tablespoon (8 g) tapioca flour

1 tablespoon (14 g) coconut oil

3 garlic cloves, minced

1½ pounds (680 g) flank steak, thinly sliced against the grain

½ teaspoon salt

¼ teaspoon black pepper

2 cups (142 g) broccoli florets

1 red bell pepper, seeded and thinly sliced

1 cup (110 g) shredded carrot

1 cup (75 g) sugar snap peas

Cooked quinoa or brown rice, for serving

Sliced scallions and sesame seeds, for garnish

—
Yield | 6 servings

In a small bowl or large measuring cup, whisk together the broth, coconut aminos, maple syrup, ginger, and tapioca flour. Set aside.

Melt the coconut oil in a wok or large skillet over medium heat. Add the garlic and stir constantly for 1 minute. Turn the heat up to high, add the steak, and season with the salt and pepper. Allow the steak to fry and crisp without stirring for 1 to 2 minutes, then stir-fry until charred and cooked to medium-rare, 4 to 5 minutes. Add the broccoli, bell pepper, carrot, and snap peas and stir-fry for 4 to 5 minutes.

Re-whisk the reserved sauce and pour it over the steak and vegetables. Cook until the sauce is thickened, 2 to 3 minutes. Serve over quinoa or rice, garnished with scallions and sesame seeds.

PRO TIP!

Throw the steak in the freezer 30 minutes before slicing. It's easier to slice the steak when it's slightly frozen.

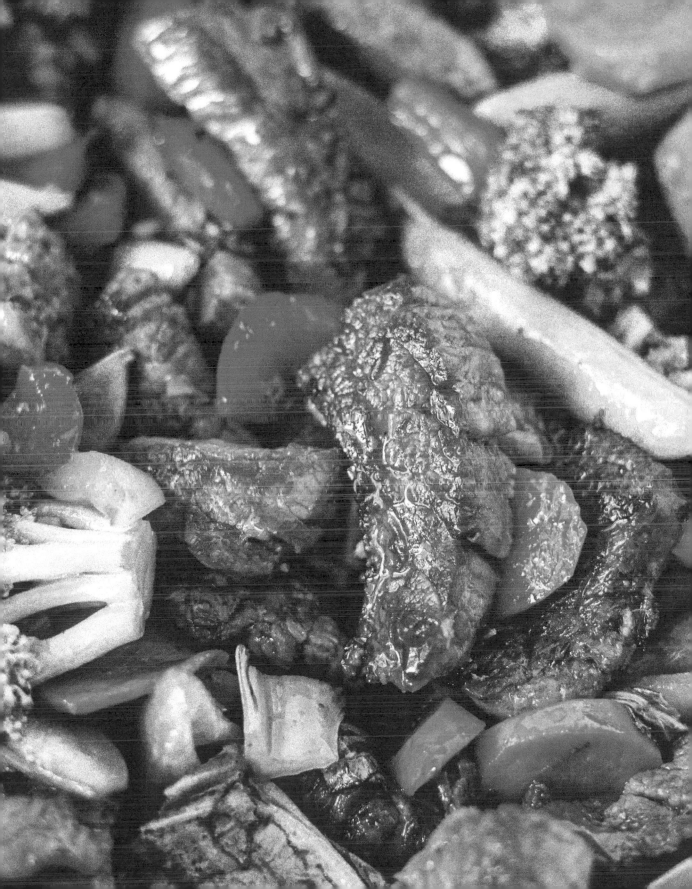

Slow Cooker Stuffed Pepper Soup

This recipe has everything I love about traditional stuffed peppers, like ground beef, tomatoes, veggies, and rice, but in a big, hearty bowl of soup. It reminds me of chili, but it's got a little less kick, a little more peppers, and a lot more rice. The peppers are full of antioxidants with strong anti-inflammatory effects.

1½ tablespoons (22 ml) olive oil

1 medium yellow onion, diced

3 garlic cloves, minced

1 pound (454 g) ground beef

4 cups (946 ml) beef broth

1 red bell pepper, seeded and diced

1 green bell pepper, seeded and diced

1 (14.5-ounce/425 g) can tomato sauce

1 (14.5-ounce/425 g) can diced tomatoes, including liquid

2 cups (390 g) long-grain white or brown rice

1 teaspoon paprika

1 teaspoon dried oregano

1 teaspoon dried dill

1 teaspoon salt

¼ teaspoon black pepper

—

Yield | 8 servings

Heat the oil in a large skillet over medium-high heat. Add the onion and cook, stirring occasionally, for 3 to 4 minutes, until soft and translucent. Add the garlic and cook for 1 to 2 more minutes, until fragrant. Add the ground beef and cook, breaking up the meat, until browned and no pink remains, 3 to 5 minutes.

Transfer the contents of the skillet to the slow cooker and add the rest of the ingredients. Stir to mix well. Cover and cook on low for 5 to 6 hours.

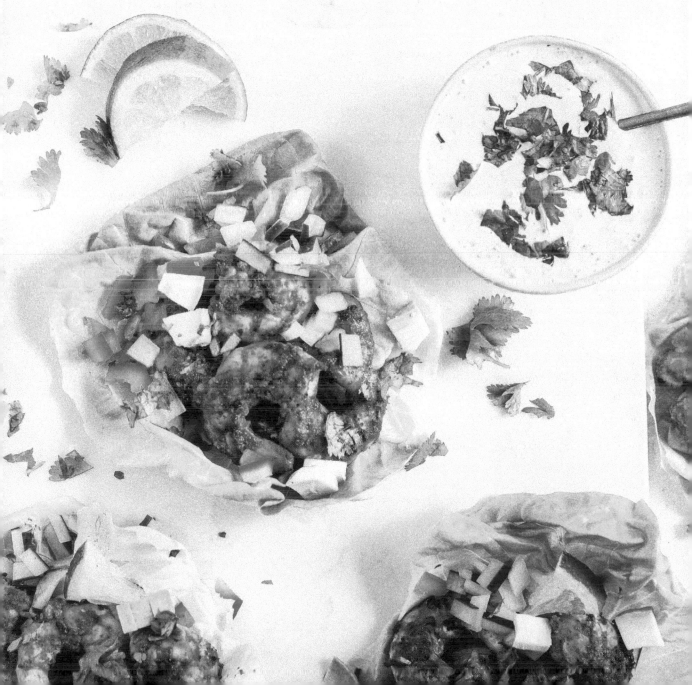

Spicy Shrimp Lettuce Wraps, page 103

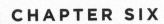

Seafood

BBQ Shrimp Tacos

If you know someone who doesn't love shrimp, let them try this recipe and I have a feeling you will change their mind! The omega-3-rich shrimp are covered in a bold, tangy BBQ sauce that's free of refined sugar. The veggies, avocado, and cilantro on top create the perfect (maybe a little messy) bite.

For the BBQ sauce:

¼ cup (61 g) canned tomato sauce

2 tablespoons (40 g) pure maple syrup

1 tablespoon (15 ml) apple cider vinegar

½ teaspoon spicy brown mustard

1 teaspoon tomato paste

2 teaspoons smoked paprika

¼ teaspoon onion powder

¼ teaspoon garlic powder

¼ teaspoon salt

For the shrimp:

2 teaspoons smoked paprika

1 teaspoon onion powder

1 teaspoon garlic powder

1 teaspoon salt

¼ teaspoon black pepper

1 pound (454 g) shrimp, peeled and deveined

2 tablespoons (28 g) coconut oil

For the tacos:

8 Two-Ingredient Grain-Free Tortillas (page 39) or store-bought grain-free tortillas

1 (1-pound/454 g) package shredded coleslaw mix

1 avocado, peeled, pitted, and diced

¼ red onion, diced

Lime wedges and chopped fresh cilantro, for garnish

—

Yield | 4 servings

To make the BBQ sauce, in a small bowl, whisk together the tomato sauce, maple syrup, apple cider vinegar, brown mustard, tomato paste, smoked paprika, onion powder, garlic powder, and salt. Set aside.

To make the shrimp, in a large bowl, combine the smoked paprika, onion powder, garlic powder, salt, and black pepper. Pat the shrimp dry and add it to the spice mixture. Toss to evenly coat.

Melt the coconut oil in a large skillet over high heat. Add the shrimp and cook for about 2 minutes on each side, until the shrimp are golden and opaque.

Add the BBQ sauce and stir to coat the shrimp in the sauce. Turn the heat down to low and allow to simmer and thicken for 3 to 5 minutes, stirring frequently. Remove from the heat.

To make the tacos, warm the tortillas in the microwave for 15 to 20 seconds, then lay them out to assemble. Put ¼ cup (20 g) of the coleslaw mix at the bottom of the tortilla and add 3 or 4 BBQ shrimp. Top with the avocado, red onion, a squeeze of lime juice, and some chopped cilantro. Roll up and enjoy.

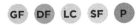

Shrimp Scampi Spaghetti Squash Boats

If you're looking for an anti-inflammatory powerhouse combo, it's spaghetti squash and shrimp. Both are packed with healthy fats, and the squash also provides vitamins A and C. This meal is also gluten- and dairy-free!

For the squash boats:

2 large spaghetti squash

2 tablespoons (30 ml) olive oil

1 teaspoon kosher salt

For the shrimp scampi:

1 pound (454 g) shrimp, peeled and deveined

2 tablespoons (30 ml) olive oil, divided

4 garlic cloves, minced, divided

½ teaspoon kosher salt

½ teaspoon crushed red pepper

4 tablespoons (55 g) ghee, divided

⅓ cup (79 ml) chicken or vegetable broth

2 tablespoons (30 ml) lemon juice (about ½ lemon)

¼ teaspoon kosher salt

2 tablespoons (8 g) minced fresh parsley, plus more for garnish

—
Yield | 4 servings

Preheat the oven to 425°F (220°C). Line a rimmed baking sheet with parchment paper or a silicone baking mat.

To make the squash boats, cut the spaghetti squash in half lengthwise, then scoop out and discard the seeds. Drizzle the cut sides with the olive oil and sprinkle with the salt. Place the squash halves, cut-sides down, on the prepared baking sheet and bake for 25 minutes.

To make the shrimp scampi, in a medium bowl, toss the shrimp with 1 tablespoon (15 ml) of the olive oil, half of the minced garlic, the salt, and the crushed red pepper.

Heat the remaining 1 tablespoon (15 ml) olive oil in a large skillet over medium heat. Add the shrimp and cook until golden brown and opaque, 1 to 2 minutes per side. Transfer the shrimp to a bowl or plate.

Melt 3 tablespoons (14 g) of the ghee in the same skillet over medium-low heat. Add the remaining garlic and cook for 1 to 2 minutes, until fragrant. Add the broth and lemon juice and deglaze the pan by scraping any cooked bits off the bottom. Cook for 5 to 6 minutes, stirring frequently so the garlic doesn't burn, until the sauce has reduced by half and thickens.

Return the shrimp to the pan and stir in the remaining 1 tablespoon (14 g) ghee, the salt, and the parsley. Stir and cook for 1 to 2 more minutes. Remove the pan from the heat and cover to keep warm.

When the spaghetti squash is done, allow it to cool briefly until it is cool enough to handle. Use a fork to shred both sides of the squash to create spaghetti strands. Scoop out all the spaghetti squash and add it to the skillet with the shrimp scampi. Toss to evenly coat. Scoop the mixture back into the empty spaghetti squash halves and place back in the oven for 8 to 10 minutes to heat through. Serve immediately, topped with more chopped parsley.

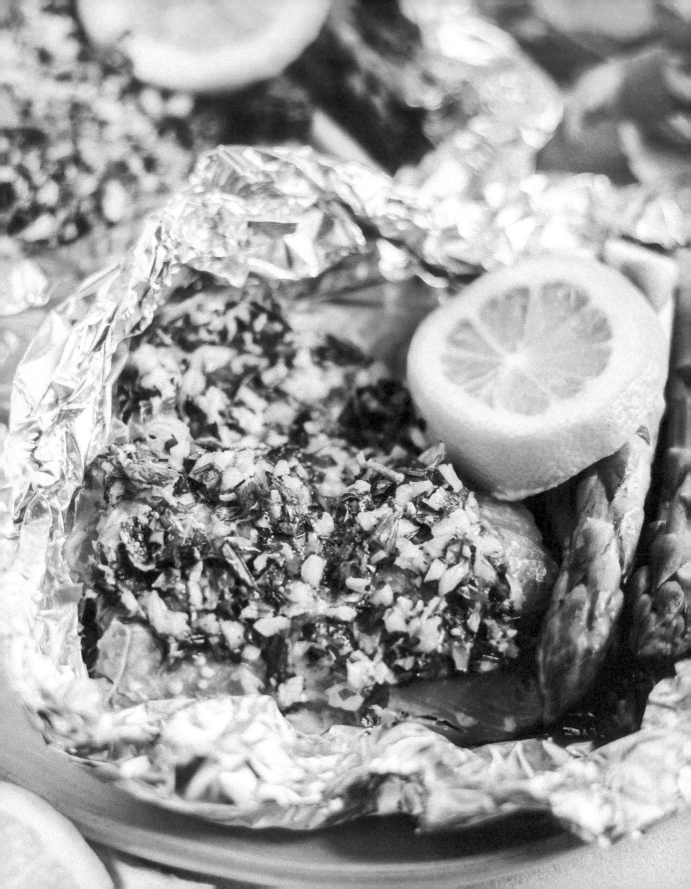

Lemon, Garlic, and Asparagus Salmon Foil Packs

Salmon is a potent source of omega-3s, which help fight inflammation and keep all the cells in your body healthy. Springtime is an especially good time to make this recipe because asparagus is at its peak, and it's loaded with antioxidants.

6 tablespoons (85 g) ghee

6 garlic cloves, minced

3 tablespoons (12 g) chopped fresh parsley

1 teaspoon chopped fresh rosemary

1 teaspoon chopped fresh thyme

4 (6-ounce/170 g) wild-caught salmon fillets

1 teaspoon salt

¼ teaspoon black pepper

2 pounds (907 g) asparagus, trimmed

3 tablespoons (45 ml) fresh lemon juice, plus 4 thin lemon slices

—

Yield | 4 servings

Preheat the oven to 400°F (200°C).

In a small bowl, combine the ghee, garlic, parsley, rosemary, and thyme and mix together with a fork.

Spread out four very large pieces of aluminum foil on your work surface. Place a salmon fillet on each sheet of foil and season with the salt and pepper. Divide the asparagus evenly next to the salmon and top each with some lemon juice and a slice of lemon. Divide the ghee and herb mixture evenly among the packets. Bring the sides of the foil up and over the contents, then, leaving some room between the salmon and foil, fold tightly to create a sealed and tented packet. Place the packets on a rimmed baking sheet.

Bake for 15 to 18 minutes, until the salmon flakes easily with a fork and reaches an internal temperature of 145°F (63°C). Carefully open the packets and serve.

> **PRO TIP!**
>
> Want to break out the grill? Heat your grill to medium-high and add the foil packets. Close the lid and grill for 10 to 15 minutes.

Shrimp Egg Roll in a Bowl

Take the insides of your favorite egg roll flavors and put them in a bowl for a simple, 15-minute meal that's full of healthy fats and veggies. Spice it up with creamy aioli and your dinner will never be the same.

For the aioli:

½ cup (115 g) paleo mayonnaise

1 tablespoon (15 g) red chile paste

1 teaspoon lime juice

1 tablespoon (15 ml) rice vinegar

2 teaspoons pure maple syrup

For the shrimp bowl:

1 pound (454 g) shrimp, peeled and deveined

Juice of 1 lime, divided

½ teaspoon salt

2 tablespoons (28 g) coconut oil, divided

2 garlic cloves, minced

1 teaspoon grated fresh ginger

1½ (1-pound/454 g) packages shredded coleslaw mix

⅓ cup (83 g) coconut aminos

1 tablespoon (20 g) pure maple syrup

¼ cup (15 g) chopped scallions

—

Yield | 5 servings

To make the aioli, in a medium bowl, whisk together all the aioli ingredients. Cover and refrigerate until ready to serve.

To make the shrimp, in a medium bowl, toss the shrimp with half of the lime juice and the salt. Melt 1 tablespoon (14 g) of the coconut oil in a large sauté pan or wok over high heat. Add the shrimp and cook for about 2 minutes on each side, until golden and opaque. Transfer to paper towels. Pour off any excess liquid from the pan.

Add the remaining 1 tablespoon (14 g) coconut oil to the pan and allow to melt over medium heat. Add the garlic and ginger and stir-fry for 1 to 2 minutes. Add the coleslaw mix, coconut aminos, maple syrup, and remaining lime juice. Stir-fry for 3 to 5 minutes, until just wilted. Return the shrimp to the pan and mix well to combine. Top with the scallions. Divide among serving bowls and drizzle with the aioli.

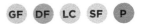

Crispy Pan-Seared Scallops with Garlic Kale

Fresh scallops are almost always available at your grocery store seafood counter, and the best news is they're usually wild-caught. When scallops are cooked properly, the outside gets crispy while the inside cuts like butter. This meal gives you anti-inflammatory compounds from the omega-3s in the scallops as well as all the nutrients in the kale.

7 cups (1656 ml) lukewarm water

¼ cup (75 g) salt

3 tablespoons (43 g) ghee, divided

1¼ pounds (567 g) sea scallops

¼ cup (59 ml) vegetable broth

2 cups (10 ounces/283 g) kale, stemmed and chopped

1 tablespoon (15 ml) lemon juice

4 garlic cloves, minced

½ teaspoon salt

Chopped fresh parsley, for garnish

—
Yield | 4 servings

Combine the lukewarm water and salt in a large bowl and stir to dissolve. Add the scallops to the brine and allow to sit for 10 minutes. Drain the scallops and rinse under cool water. Pat both sides dry with paper towels.

Melt 1 tablespoon (15 g) of the ghee in a large cast-iron skillet over high heat. Add the scallops and gently press them down with the back of a spatula to help create a crust. Sear without moving them until the bottoms are a rich golden brown, 2 to 2½ minutes. Add another 1 tablespoon (15 g) ghee to the pan, then flip each scallop over. Tilt the pan and use a spoon to scoop the melted ghee over the scallops to baste them. Cook for another 1 to 2 minutes on the second side. The scallops should be opaque and firm to the touch, with an internal temperature of 145°F (63°C). Use tongs to transfer the cooked scallops to a plate lined with paper towels.

Turn the heat to low and add the vegetable broth to the pan to deglaze it, scraping the little bits off the bottom of the pan. Add the remaining 1 tablespoon (15 g) ghee and allow it to melt. Add the kale and lemon juice and cook, stirring frequently, until soft and wilted, 3 to 4 minutes. Add the garlic and salt and cook for about 1 minute, until fragrant. Return the scallops to the pan and turn a few times to coat in the garlic and lemon sauce. Garnish with parsley.

Sheet Pan Almond-Crusted Tilapia and Veggies

You get double omega-3s in this recipe with the tilapia and almonds. The crust is crunchy and flavorful and the veggies are crispy, and it all cooks up to perfection in one pan!

For the veggies:

2 large carrots, peeled and thinly sliced

3½ cups (249 g) chopped broccoli

1 yellow squash, halved lengthwise and thinly sliced crosswise

2 tablespoons (30 ml) olive oil

1 teaspoon garlic powder

1 teaspoon salt

¼ teaspoon black pepper

For the almond- crusted tilapia:

1 cup (145 g) raw, unsalted almonds

2 large eggs

¾ cup (84 g) almond flour

¼ cup (32 g) tapioca flour

1 teaspoon dried dill

½ teaspoon paprika

½ teaspoon salt

4 (4-ounce/113 g) tilapia fillets

Lemon wedges, for garnish

—
Yield | 4 servings

Preheat the oven 425°F (220°C). Line a rimmed baking sheet with aluminum foil.

To make the veggies, combine the carrots, broccoli, and squash on the prepared baking sheet. Drizzle with the olive oil and sprinkle with the garlic powder, salt, and pepper. Toss to coat, then spread out the veggies in a single layer. Bake for 20 minutes.

While the veggies are roasting, prepare the tilapia. Put the almonds in a food processor and pulse for 20 to 30 seconds until the almonds are broken up into tiny pieces. Transfer to a medium bowl. In a separate medium bowl, beat the eggs. In a third medium bowl, whisk together the almond flour, tapioca flour, dill, paprika, and salt.

When the veggies are done roasting, remove the baking sheet from the oven and push all the vegetables to one side.

Create an assembly line with the three bowls and the baking sheet. Pat one tilapia fillet dry and dip it into the almond flour mixture, then into the egg wash, and then into the crushed almonds, pressing to help them adhere. Place the coated fillet on the empty side of the baking sheet. Repeat with the remaining fillets. Bake for 11 to 13 minutes, until the vegetables are fork-tender and the tilapia is cooked through and golden brown. Serve right away with a squeeze of lemon juice.

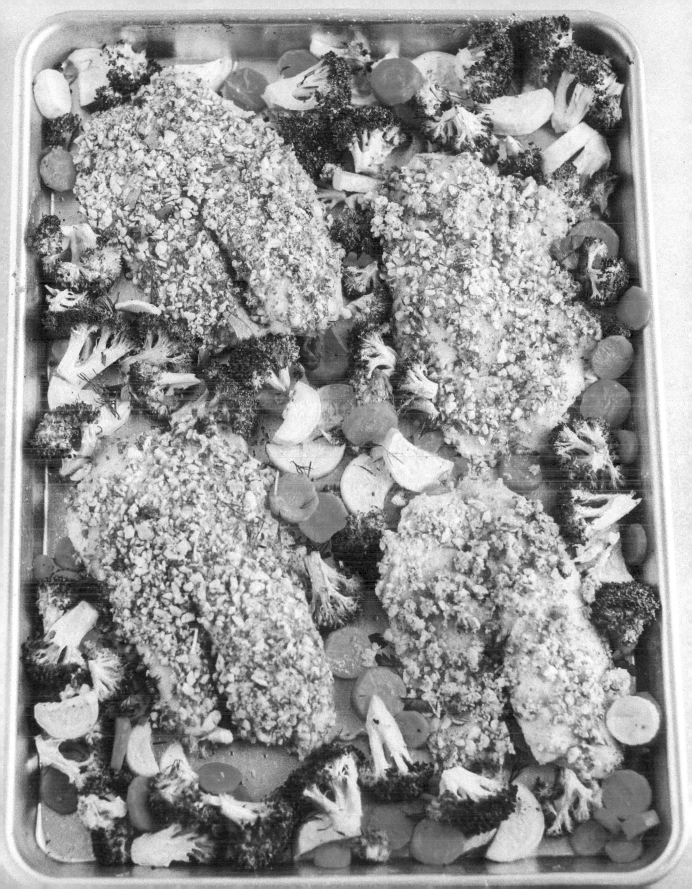

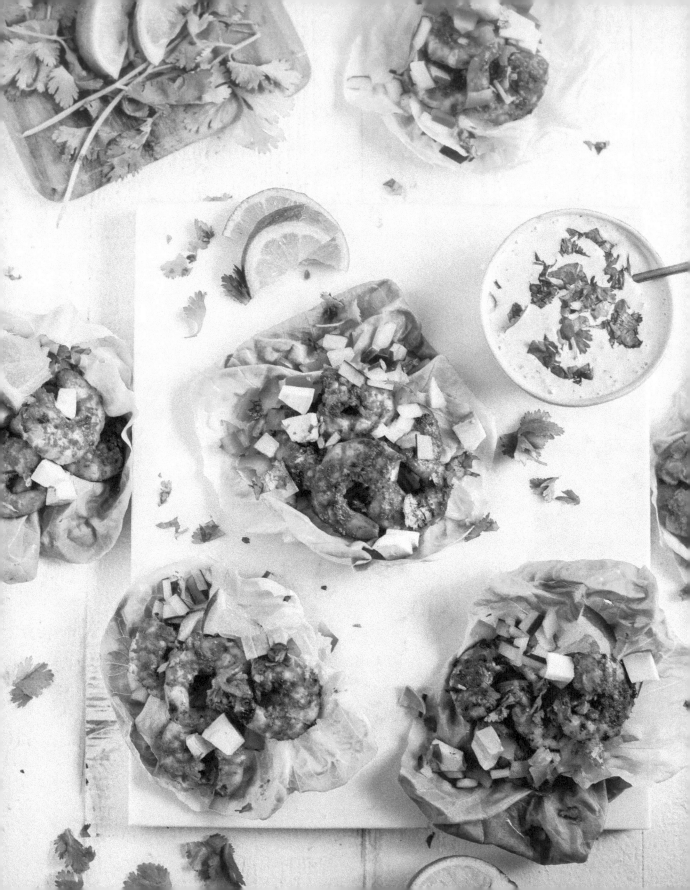

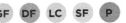

Spicy Shrimp Lettuce Wraps

Shrimp are high in omega-3s, and that makes them an amazing protein for fighting inflammation. We're adding paprika and cayenne pepper to take the anti-inflammatory level up a notch and give this meal the kick you need to spice up your weekday. Did I mention the whole recipe takes only 20 minutes from start to finish? That's an A+ meal in my book!

For the creamy cilantro sauce:

⅓ cup (75 g) paleo mayonnaise

¼ cup (58 ml) well-shaken canned full-fat coconut milk

Juice of ½ lime

¼ cup (8 g) packed chopped fresh cilantro

1 garlic clove, minced

½ teaspoon salt

For the spicy shrimp:

1 tablespoon (8 g) smoked paprika

1 teaspoon chili powder

½ teaspoon ground cumin

½ teaspoon salt

¼ teaspoon cayenne pepper

¼ teaspoon garlic powder

1 pound (454 g) shrimp, peeled and deveined

Juice of ½ lime

1 tablespoon (2 g) chopped fresh cilantro

1 tablespoon (14 g) coconut oil

For the lettuce wraps:

8 butter lettuce leaves

1 red bell pepper, seeded and thinly sliced

1 cucumber, thinly sliced

¼ red onion, thinly sliced

1 avocado, peeled, pitted, and diced

3 tablespoons (6 g) chopped fresh cilantro

—

Yield | 4 servings

To make the cilantro sauce, in a medium bowl, whisk together all the cilantro sauce ingredients. (Alternatively, you can blend everything in a food processor for 1 to 2 minutes.) Cover and refrigerate until ready to serve.

To make the shrimp, combine the paprika, chili powder, cumin, salt, cayenne, and garlic powder in a small bowl. Put the shrimp in a medium bowl and add the lime juice, cilantro, and spice mix. Toss to thoroughly coat.

Melt the coconut oil in a medium skillet over medium heat. Add the shrimp and cook until golden and opaque, 1 to 2 minutes per side.

To assemble each lettuce wrap, stack 2 lettuce leaves and add a spoonful of the shrimp in the center. Top with some bell pepper, cucumber, onion, avocado, cilantro, and sauce. Roll up and serve.

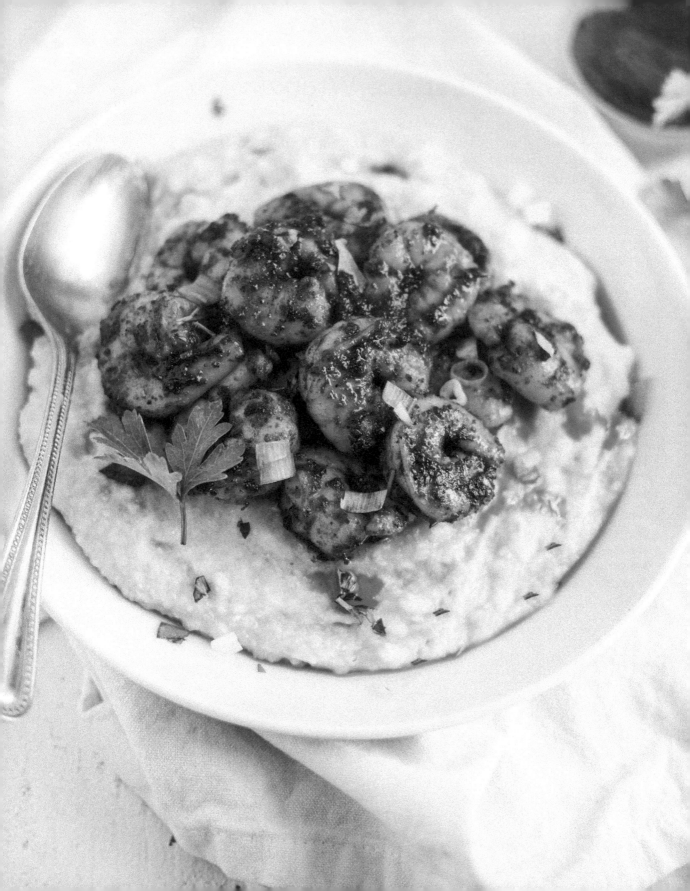

Chipotle Shrimp and Grits

Shrimp and grits originated as a breakfast dish, often called "breakfast shrimp," and has since transformed into a dish served around the world as an entree or brunch special. This recipe takes the dairy and cheese out of the grits by swapping in nutritional yeast and creamy coconut milk. The omega-3 fatty acids from the shrimp are a key player in reducing inflammation naturally.

For the grits:

1 (13.5-ounce/383 g) can full-fat coconut milk

2⅓ cups (550 ml) chicken broth

1½ teaspoons salt

1 cup (140 g) stone-ground grits

2 garlic cloves, minced

⅔ cup (156 ml) unsweetened nondairy milk

¼ cup (55 g) ghee or coconut oil

⅓ cup (33 g) nutritional yeast

¼ teaspoon black pepper

For the chipotle shrimp:

1 tablespoon (8 g) smoked paprika

2 teaspoons chili powder

1 teaspoon chipotle powder

1 teaspoon ground cumin

1 teaspoon garlic powder

1 teaspoon dried oregano

½ teaspoon ground coriander

½ teaspoon salt

1 pound (454 g) shrimp, peeled and deveined

1 tablespoon (14 g) coconut oil

Chopped fresh parsley or scallions, for garnish

—

Yield | 5 servings

To make the grits, in a medium saucepan, combine the coconut milk, chicken broth, and salt. Bring to a boil over high heat, then slowly whisk in the grits and garlic. Reduce the heat to medium-low, cover, and simmer for 20 minutes, whisking frequently.

To make the shrimp, combine all the chipotle seasonings in a medium bowl. Pat the shrimp dry and add it to the seasoning mixture. Toss to evenly coat.

Melt the coconut oil in a medium sauté pan over medium-high heat. Add the shrimp and cook for about 2 minutes on each side, until golden and opaque. Transfer the shrimp to paper towels.

When the grits are done simmering, remove from the heat and add the nondairy milk, ghee, nutritional yeast, and pepper and stir to combine. Transfer the grits to a large bowl and top with the chipotle shrimp. Garnish with parsley or scallions.

ADD IT!

Feel free to use quick-cooking grits; just take a look at the package directions for the correct cook time. It's usually around 5 minutes.

Gluten-Free Crispy Crab Cakes

When I used to think of crab cakes, I'd think of my sister ordering them on vacation anytime we'd go out to eat. It didn't cross my mind to make them at home, but they're a simple recipe that makes an amazing weeknight meal. If you can find real crabmeat rather than imitation, it'll take this recipe to the next flavor level. It includes so many healthy fats!

For the aioli:

½ cup (120 g) paleo mayonnaise

1 teaspoon Cajun seasoning

1 teaspoon hot sauce

1 teaspoon lemon juice

For the crab cakes:

1 pound (454 g) jumbo (or traditional) lump crabmeat, shredded

½ green bell pepper, seeded and finely chopped

⅓ cup (37 g) almond flour

¼ cup (60 g) paleo mayonnaise

1 large egg

1 tablespoon (15 ml) hot sauce

1 tablespoon (16 g) coconut aminos

2 teaspoons Dijon mustard

2 teaspoons lemon juice

1 tablespoon (4 g) minced fresh parsley, plus more for garnish

1 tablespoon (14 g) coconut oil

—
Yield | 4 servings

To make the aioli, in a small bowl, whisk together the aioli ingredients. Cover and refrigerate until ready to serve.

To make the crab cakes, in a large bowl, combine the crabmeat, green pepper, and almond flour until completely coated. In a medium bowl, whisk together the mayo, egg, hot sauce, coconut aminos, mustard, lemon juice, and parsley. Add this mixture to the crab mixture and stir well to combine. Divide the mixture into 8 equals parts and gently form into patties, being careful not to overwork.

Melt the coconut oil in a large skillet over medium heat. Working in batches if necessary, add the crab cakes and press down gently with the back of a spatula to help form a crust. Cook the patties for 3 minutes without moving them, then flip and cook for 3 minutes on the other side, until browned and heated through. Serve with the aioli.

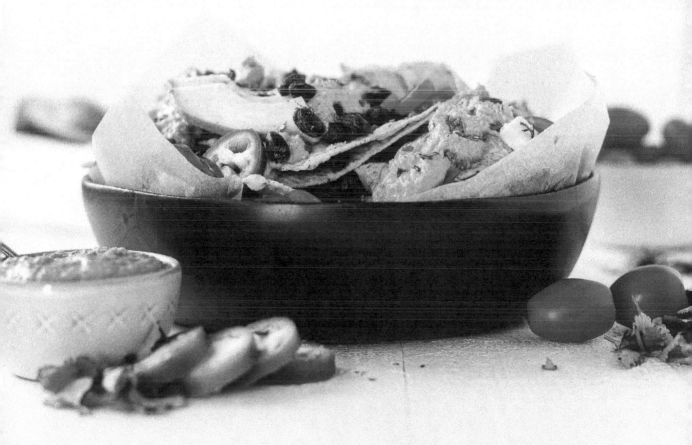

CHAPTER EIGHT

Meatless Meals
and Sides

Spicy Black Bean Nachos with Cashew Queso, page 123

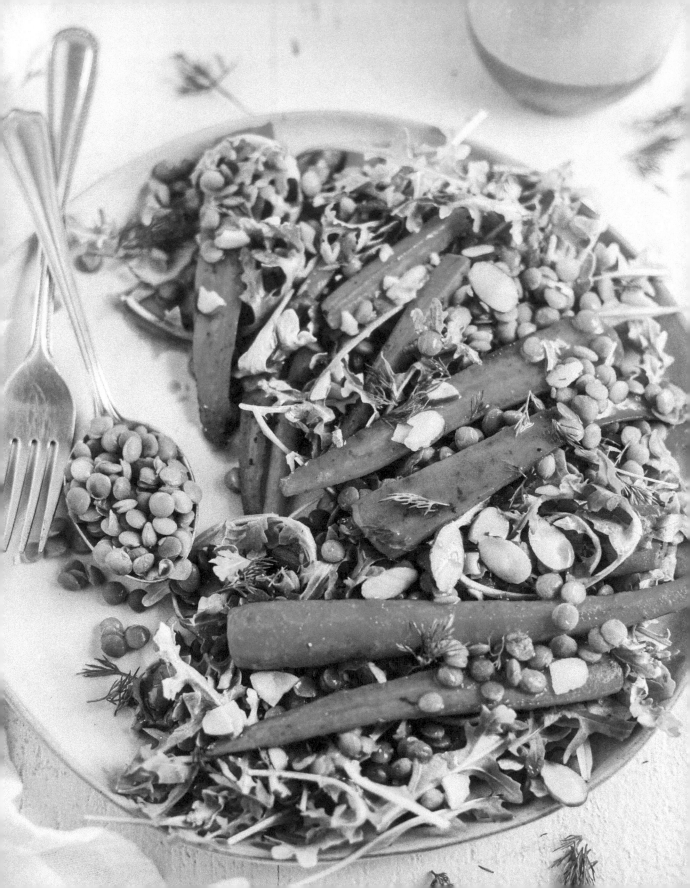

Roasted Carrot and Lentil Salad with Tahini Dressing

You're going to want to put tahini dressing on everything after you taste this recipe! The sugars in the carrots come out when they're roasted, so this recipe is a little sweet, a little peppery, and a little crunchy.

For the salad:

¾ cup (144 g) red or green lentils, rinsed

8 medium carrots, peeled and halved lengthwise

1 tablespoon (15 ml) olive oil

1 teaspoon paprika

½ teaspoon salt

¼ teaspoon black pepper

2 cups (40 g) arugula

Sliced almonds, for topping

Chopped fresh dill, for garnish (optional)

For the tahini dressing:

3 tablespoons (45 g) tahini

2 tablespoons (30 ml) balsamic vinegar

½ cup (118 ml) olive oil

1 garlic clove, minced

¼ teaspoon salt

2 teaspoons pure maple syrup

—

Yield | 2 servings

Preheat the oven to 425°F (220°C). Line a rimmed baking sheet with aluminum foil or a silicone baking mat.

To make the salad, put the lentils in a medium saucepan and cover with about 3 inches (7.5 cm) water. Cover the pan and bring to a boil over high heat. Uncover, reduce the heat to medium-low, and simmer until the lentils are tender, 20 to 25 minutes. Once cooked, drain any remaining water and set aside to cool.

Meanwhile, put the carrots on the prepared baking sheet and drizzle with the olive oil. Sprinkle with the paprika, salt, and pepper and stir to coat. Spread out in a single layer and bake for 22 to 24 minutes, stirring halfway through. The carrots should be fork-tender and golden brown.

To make the dressing, combine all the tahini dressing ingredients in a jar with a lid and shake well (or whisk together in a small bowl).

Put the arugula in a serving bowl and top with the lentils, roasted carrots, and sliced almonds, then drizzle with the tahini dressing. Garnish with fresh dill, if desired.

ADD IT!

If you don't like the peppery taste of arugula, you can swap it out for mixed field greens or baby spinach.

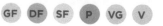

Easy Butternut Squash Soup

Thick and creamy is the best way to describe this velvety smooth soup. You will think you've been transported to a quaint New England cottage, sipping on butternut squash soup, and fighting inflammation at the same time, while the leaves slowly change to a colorful fall hue. This one freezes well, so stock up on butternut squash when you can!

Nonstick cooking spray

1 medium butternut squash

3 tablespoons (45 ml) olive oil, divided

1 teaspoon sea salt, plus more to taste

3 cups (710 ml) chicken broth, vegetable broth, or bone broth

1 yellow onion, diced

3 tablespoons (60 g) pure maple syrup

1 teaspoon ground cinnamon (optional)

½ teaspoon ground nutmeg (optional)

—

Yield | 5 servings

Preheat the oven to 400°F (200°C). Coat a rimmed baking sheet with nonstick cooking spray.

Peel the butternut squash using a vegetable peeler. Cut off the ends and cut the squash in half lengthwise. Scoop out the seeds, then cut the squash into 1-inch (2.5 cm) chunks. Spread out the chunks on the prepared baking sheet, toss with 2 tablespoons (30 ml) of the olive oil, and sprinkle with the salt. Roast for 40 minutes, stirring halfway through, until fork-tender.

Heat the remaining 1 tablespoon (15 ml) olive oil in a large Dutch oven or stockpot over medium heat. Add the onion and cook until it is translucent and starts to turn golden, 2 to 3 minutes. Add the roasted squash and broth and bring to a simmer over medium-high heat. Simmer for 10 minutes. Using an immersion blender, mix the soup until it's smooth and creamy. (Alternatively, transfer the soup, in batches if necessary, to a countertop blender and blend. Be sure to remove the center cap from the blender lid and hold a kitchen towel over the hole to allow steam to escape. Return the soup to the pot.)

Stir in the maple syrup and spices, if desired.

Black Bean and Sweet Potato Enchiladas

Black beans and sweet potatoes make a hearty filling for a meatless enchilada. Customize this fiber-filled fiesta with all your favorite toppings for a complete meal in one casserole.

Nonstick cooking spray

2 tablespoons (28 g) coconut oil

1 large or 2 medium sweet potatoes, peeled and cut into 1-inch (2.5 cm) pieces

½ medium yellow onion, chopped

1 medium bell pepper (any color), seeded and diced

2 garlic cloves, minced

1 teaspoon ground cumin

½ teaspoon garlic powder

½ teaspoon onion powder

½ teaspoon salt

¼ teaspoon black pepper

1 (15-ounce/432 g) can black beans, rinsed and drained

3 tablespoons (6 g) minced fresh cilantro, plus more for garnish (optional)

1 (10-ounce/283 g) can no-sugar-added red enchilada sauce, divided

8 corn tortillas or Two-Ingredient Grain-Free Tortillas (page 39)

Chopped jalapeños, chopped avocado, and/or chopped tomatoes, for garnish (optional)

—

Yield | 4 servings

Preheat the oven to 350°F (180°C). Coat a 9 × 13-inch (23 × 33 cm) baking pan with nonstick cooking spray.

Melt the coconut oil in a deep sauté pan over medium heat. Add the sweet potatoes and cook, stirring occasionally, for 10 to 12 minutes, until fork-tender and a little brown and crispy. Add the onion and bell pepper and cook for another 2 to 3 minutes. Add the garlic, cumin, garlic powder, onion powder, salt, and pepper. Stir and cook for another minute. Add the black beans, cilantro, and 3 tablespoons (45 g) of the enchilada sauce and stir well to combine. Remove the pan from the heat.

Pour ½ cup (120 g) of the remaining enchilada sauce in a shallow bowl. Warm the tortillas in the microwave for 15 to 20 seconds, until soft and pliable. Dip each tortilla in the enchilada sauce, then spoon ¼ cup (56 g) of the sweet potato and black bean mixture into the tortilla. Fold the tortilla over the filling and roll it up. Place the enchilada seam-down in the prepared baking dish. Repeat to fill all the tortillas, lining up the enchiladas in the pan.

Top the enchiladas with the remaining sauce. Bake for 15 minutes, or until the sauce is bubbling. Let everyone top their enchiladas however they like.

Crispy Chickpea Caesar Salad

This recipe was one of the first I knew I wanted to put in this book. I love the idea of swapping chickpeas for chicken to make a vegetarian dish. You don't need dairy for the easy dressing, either!

For the salad:

1 (15-ounce/432 g) can chickpeas, rinsed and drained

2 tablespoons (30 ml) extra-virgin olive oil, divided

1 teaspoon smoked paprika

½ teaspoon garlic powder

½ teaspoon salt, divided

¼ teaspoon black pepper

3 cups (201 g) chopped kale, stems removed and leaves torn or cut into thin pieces

1 tablespoon (15 ml) lemon juice

For the dressing:

½ cup (118 ml) lemon juice (about 2 lemons)

⅓ cup (79 ml) extra-virgin olive oil

⅓ cup (33 g) nutritional yeast

2 garlic cloves, minced

2 tablespoons (8 g) chopped fresh parsley

2 tablespoons (30 g) tahini

1 tablespoon (12 g) Dijon mustard

2 teaspoons coconut aminos

1 teaspoon pure maple syrup

½ teaspoon salt

¼ teaspoon black pepper

3 to 4 tablespoons (45 to 60 ml) water

—

Yield | 6 servings

Preheat the oven to 425°F (220°C). Line a rimmed baking sheet with aluminum foil.

To make the salad, on the prepared baking sheet, toss the chickpeas with 1 tablespoon (15 ml) of the olive oil and the smoked paprika, garlic powder, ¼ teaspoon of the salt, and the pepper. Spread them out in a single layer and bake for 25 minutes, stirring halfway through.

Meanwhile, put the kale in a large bowl. Drizzle with the lemon juice, remaining 1 tablespoon (15 ml) olive oil, and remaining ¼ teaspoon salt. Use your hands to massage the kale until the leaves start to soften and wilt.

To make the dressing, combine all the dressing ingredients except for the water in a food processor. Blend on high until smooth. Add 3 tablespoons (45 ml) water and blend again. If it's still too thick, add 1 more tablespoon (15 ml) water and blend again.

Drizzle half of the dressing over the kale and mix well. When the chickpeas are done, add them to the salad and drizzle with the rest of the dressing before serving.

ADD IT!

Want a little kick? Add ¼ teaspoon cayenne pepper to your chickpeas for a spicy twist!

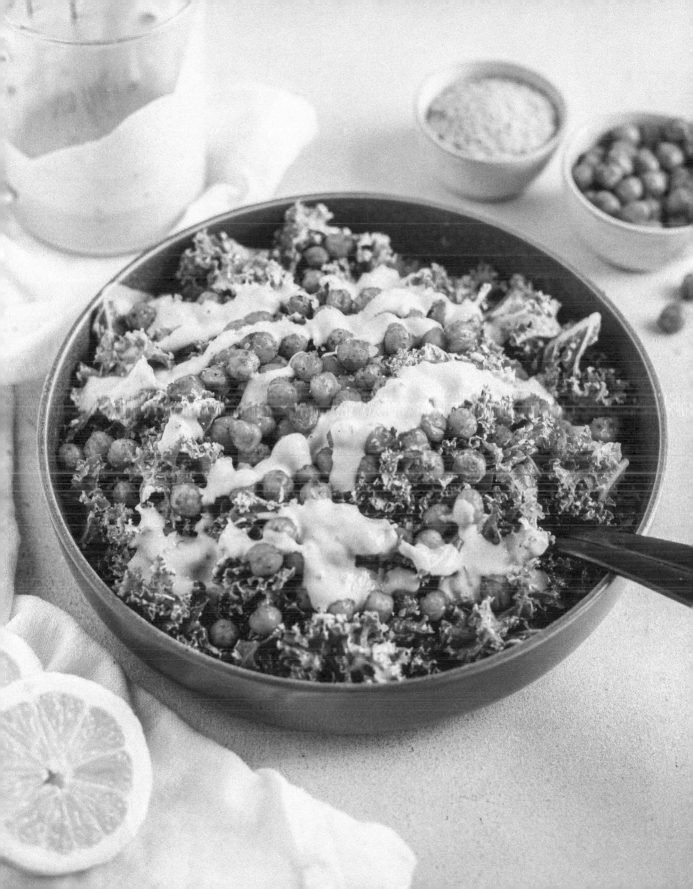

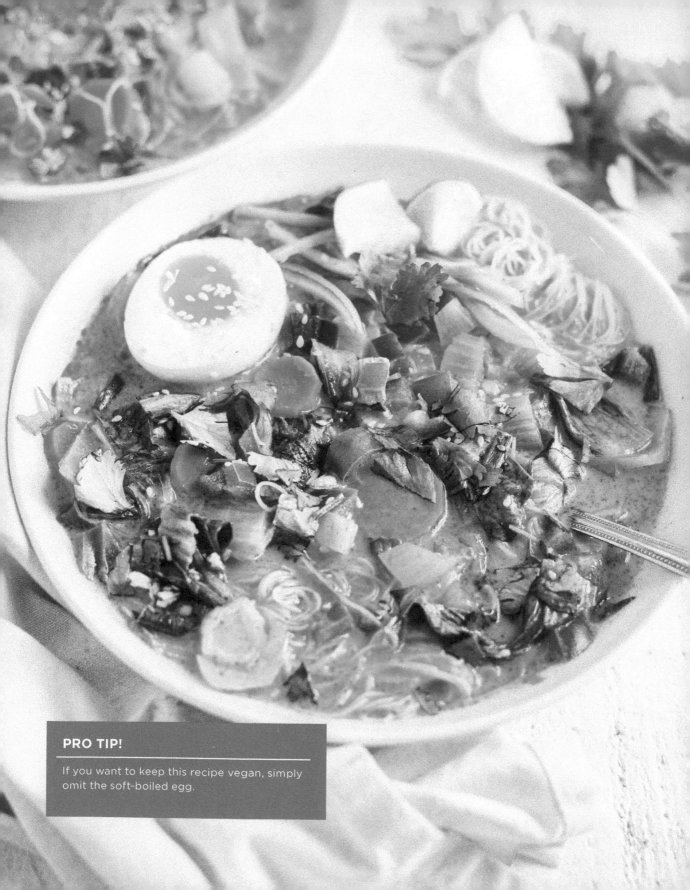

PRO TIP!

If you want to keep this recipe vegan, simply omit the soft-boiled egg.

Veggie-Filled Coconut Noodle Soup with a Soft-Boiled Egg

Cruciferous vegetables, like bok choy, are a great source of phytonutrients, which are plant-based compounds that help lower inflammation. Chinese cabbage looks like a cross between celery and lettuce, and it makes a special appearance in this soup along with other inflammation-fighting ingredients like bell pepper, ginger, and carrot. This recipe cooks quickly, so make sure you have all the ingredients prepped and chopped before starting.

2 large eggs, cold

1 tablespoon (14 g) coconut oil

3 garlic cloves, minced

2 teaspoons grated fresh ginger

3 tablespoons (45 g) red curry paste

1 bell pepper (any color), seeded and thinly sliced

2 medium carrots, thinly sliced

2 baby bok choy, thinly sliced, white stalks and green leaves reserved separately

4 cups (946 ml) vegetable broth

1 (13.5-ounce/383 g) can full-fat coconut milk

1 tablespoon (16 g) coconut aminos

2 teaspoons pure maple syrup

1 teaspoon salt

4 ounces (115 g) package vermicelli noodles

½ medium red onion, thinly sliced

¼ cup (16 g) chopped fresh cilantro

Juice of 1 lime

—

Yield | 4 servings

Pour 1 inch (2.5 cm) of water into a small saucepan and bring to a boil over high heat. Add the eggs straight from the refrigerator, cover, and allow to boil for 6 minutes. While it's boiling, fill a medium bowl with water and ice cubes. After 6 minutes, remove the eggs from the water with a slotted spoon and immediately place in the ice bath to stop cooking. Set aside to cool.

Melt the coconut oil in a deep sauté pan or stockpot over medium heat. Add the garlic, ginger, and red curry paste and stir well to heat for 1 to 2 minutes. Add the bell pepper, carrots, and white bok choy stalks. Add the vegetable broth and turn the heat up to medium-high. Bring the mixture to a boil, then reduce the heat to medium-low and simmer for 4 to 5 minutes, until the carrots are tender.

Add the coconut milk, coconut aminos, maple syrup, and salt and stir well to combine. Add the green bok choy leaves, stir, and allow to wilt for 1 to 2 minutes. Add the noodles and cook for 3 minutes, or until al dente.

Remove the eggs from the ice bath and peel.

To serve, ladle the soup into bowls and top with sliced red onion, chopped cilantro, and a squeeze of lime juice. Carefully cut the eggs in half lengthwise and place one half on top of each bowl.

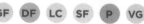

Crispy Brussels Sprouts

Every time we visit my parents, my dad makes these crispy Brussels sprouts. It's become a family staple! This recipe reminds me of home and family gatherings. They can be served as a healthy appetizer before your meal or as a simple side to go with chicken or steak.

For the Brussels sprouts:

2 pounds (910 g) Brussels sprouts, trimmed and halved lengthwise (or quartered if large)

2 tablespoons (30 ml) olive oil

1 teaspoon garlic powder

1 teaspoon salt

½ teaspoon black pepper

For the chipotle aioli:

1 cup (225 g) paleo mayonnaise

4 canned chipotles in adobo sauce

2 teaspoons lime juice

¼ teaspoon salt

⅛ teaspoon black pepper

—

Yield | 6 to 8 servings

Preheat the oven to 400°F (200°C). Line a rimmed baking sheet with parchment paper or a silicone baking mat.

To make the Brussels sprouts, put the sprouts on the prepared baking sheet and drizzle with the olive oil. Sprinkle with the garlic powder, salt, and pepper and toss to coat. Spread out in a single layer and roast for 30 to 35 minutes, until the Brussels sprouts are fork-tender and browned and crispy.

To make the aioli, combine all the aioli ingredients in a food processor or a small blender. Blend on high for 1 to 2 minutes, until the mixture is smooth and creamy. Serve the Brussels sprouts with the aioli.

PRO TIP!

Cans of chipotles in adobo sauce are usually found in the international section of the grocery store. If you have leftovers, this condiment is great on sandwiches, burgers, tacos, and more.

ADD IT!

If you want fried Brussels sprouts, fill a Dutch oven with few inches (7.5 cm) avocado oil and let it get really hot, right before smoking. Work in three or four batches to fry the Brussels sprouts for 3 to 5 minutes, or until they start to crisp and brown. Use a slotted spoon to transfer them to a paper towel to cool and drain.

Caramelized Onion and Black Bean Burgers

This recipe starts by caramelizing onions to get a deep, rich flavor. It's what makes these black bean burgers unique! The fiber and antioxidants from the beans are great for combating inflammation. Serve on your favorite gluten-free bun with lettuce and tomato, in a lettuce wrap, or over a salad.

1 tablespoon (14 g) coconut oil

1½ large yellow onions, sliced

½ bell pepper (any color), seeded and chopped

3 garlic cloves, minced

3 tablespoons (24 g) tapioca flour

2 tablespoons (32 g) coconut aminos

2 tablespoons (28 g) paleo mayonnaise

1 teaspoons ground cumin

1 teaspoonsmoked paprika

½ teaspoon chili powder

½ teaspoon salt

¼ teaspoon black pepper

2 (15-ounce/432 g) cans black beans, rinsed and drained

—

Yield | 6 servings

Preheat the oven to 375°F (190°C). Line a rimmed baking sheet with parchment paper or a silicone baking mat.

Melt the coconut oil in a medium saucepan over medium heat. Add the onion and cook, stirring frequently, for 12 to 15 minutes, until they become very soft and start to caramelize. Transfer half of the onion to a plate and cover with aluminum foil to keep warm. Add the bell pepper and garlic to the pan and cook for another 2 to 3 minutes, until soft. Transfer the contents of the pan to a food processor and add the tapioca flour, coconut aminos, mayo, cumin, smoked paprika, chili powder, salt, and pepper. Pulse everything together until combined. Add three-quarters of the beans (about 1½ cans) and pulse a few times until just combined. Add the remaining black beans and stir into the mixture, leaving them whole.

For each burger, scoop out ⅓ cup (100 g) of the mixture and form a patty. Place on the prepared baking sheet. Bake for 12 minutes, flipping halfway through.

Serve with the reserved caramelized onions on top.

Marinated Chickpea and Brussels Sprouts Greek Salad

I love to use Brussels sprouts as the base of salads rather than spinach or lettuce. This cruciferous vegetable contains antioxidants and compounds that fight inflammation. The chickpeas add fiber, and they're marinated to give extra Greek flavor. This salad is great to make ahead of time because Brussels sprouts hold up well in the fridge.

For the marinated chickpeas:

1 (15-ounce/432 g)can chickpeas, rinsed and drained

⅓ cup (79 ml) olive oil

1 teaspoon chopped fresh thyme

1 teaspoon chopped fresh oregano

½ teaspoon salt

½ teaspoon crushed red pepper

For the Greek salad:

1½ pounds (680 g) Brussels sprouts, trimmed

2 cups (270 g) diced cucumber (about 1 medium cucumber)

1 cup (180 g) cherry tomatoes, quartered

½ cup (50 g) kalamata olives, halved

1 medium avocado, peeled, pitted, and diced

½ medium red onion, diced

For the creamy Greek dressing:

¼ cup (59 ml) olive oil

3 tablespoons (45 ml) red wine vinegar

1 tablespoon (15 ml) lemon juice

1 teaspoon Dijon mustard

1 small shallot, minced

2 teaspoons paleo mayonnaise

1 garlic clove, minced

1 tablespoon (4 g) chopped fresh parsley

1 teaspoon chopped fresh oregano

½ teaspoon salt

¼ teaspoon black pepper

—

Yield | 8 to 10 servings

To make the marinated chickpeas, in a medium bowl, toss the chickpeas with the olive oil, thyme, oregano, salt, and crushed red pepper. Set aside to marinate for at least 10 minutes while you prepare the rest of the salad.

To make the Greek salad, put the Brussels sprouts in a food processor and pulse a few times to chop, leaving a few large pieces. Alternatively, you could thinly slice the Brussels sprouts with a knife. Transfer the Brussels sprouts to a large bowl and add the cucumber, tomatoes, olives, avocado, and red onion.

To make the dressing, strain the chickpeas over a small bowl, reserving the liquid. Add the chickpeas to the salad. Transfer the strained oil to a jar with a lid, add the additional ¼ cup (59 ml) olive oil and remaining dressing ingredients, and shake well (or whisk everything together in the small bowl).

Pour the dressing over the salad and toss well to coat.

ADD IT!

If you don't want to use Brussels sprouts, you can substitute spinach or kale massaged with olive oil.

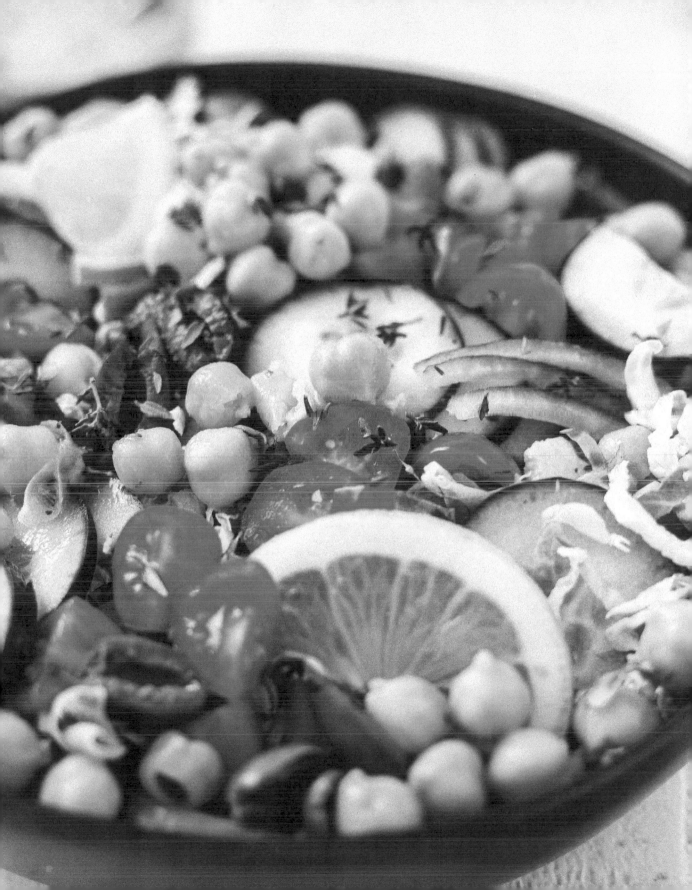

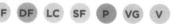
Curry Cauliflower Bowls

This recipe shows that you need never feel stuck for ways to add more vegetables to your diet. I hope you will be inspired to add any vegetable you have on hand to this dish! It's easy to customize with inflammation-fighting ingredients you have on hand, like leafy greens, beans, or potatoes.

2 tablespoons (28 g) coconut oil

1 medium yellow onion, diced

2 to 3 garlic cloves, minced

1 tablespoon (8 g) grated fresh ginger or 2 teaspoons ground ginger

1 teaspoon ground coriander

1 teaspoon salt

¼ cup (60 g) red curry paste

3 medium carrots, peeled and thinly sliced

4 cups (400 g) cauliflower florets (about 1 head of cauliflower)

¾ cup (177 ml) vegetable broth

1 (15-ounce/432 g) can chickpeas, rinsed and drained

1 (13.5-ounce/383 g) can full-fat coconut milk

4 cups (120 g) baby spinach, packed

2 tablespoons (32 g) coconut aminos

1 tablespoon (15 ml) lime juice

Cooked rice, for serving

Chopped fresh cilantro and chopped peanuts or cashews, for topping

—
Yield | 4 servings

Melt the coconut oil in a large skillet over medium heat. Add the onion and cook, stirring occasionally, until soft and translucent, 5 to 6 minutes. Add the garlic and cook for 1 to 2 minutes, until fragrant. Add the ginger, coriander, salt, and red curry paste, stir to combine, and cook for another 1 to 2 minutes. Add the carrots and cauliflower and stir to combine. Allow the vegetables to cook for 4 to 5 minutes, until a bit soft, but not fork-tender. Add the vegetable broth and chickpeas. Cover, turn the heat to high, and bring to a boil, then reduce the heat to low and simmer for 8 to 10 minutes. The cauliflower should be fork-tender at this point.

Add the coconut milk, spinach, coconut aminos, and lime juice and stir until combined and creamy and the spinach is wilted. Serve with white rice, topped with chopped cilantro and nuts.

ADD IT!

You can swap out the chickpeas for 1 medium sweet potato, peeled and diced small. It's another great anti-inflammatory option, full of vitamin A.

Moroccan Lentil Stew with Mashed Potatoes

If you've never made a Moroccan-inspired dish, get ready to be wowed! The punch of spices is warm and welcoming, while all the veggies fight off inflammation. This is the true definition of eating the rainbow!

For the mashed potatoes:

2 pounds (907 g) russet potatoes, peeled and quartered

½ cup (115 g) coconut cream

2 tablespoons (28 g) ghee

1 teaspoon sea salt

¼ teaspoon black pepper

3 to 5 tablespoons (45 to 75 ml) unsweetened nondairy milk

For the lentil stew:

3 tablespoons (45 ml) olive oil

3 medium carrots, peeled and diced small

1 medium yellow onion, diced small

2 celery stalks, diced small

4 garlic cloves, minced

2 tablespoons (15 g) smoked paprika

1½ teaspoons ground cumin

1 teaspoon ground turmeric

¾ teaspoon ground cinnamon

1 teaspoon salt

¼ teaspoon black pepper

4 cups (946 ml) vegetable broth

1¼ cups (240 g) red lentils, rinsed

2 tablespoons (30 ml) fresh lemon juice

1 cup (67 g) chopped kale

Fresh cilantro or parsley leaves, for garnish

—

Yield | 6 servings

To make the mashed potatoes, put the potatoes in a large pot and cover with water. Bring to a boil over high heat, then reduce to low and simmer for 15 to 18 minutes, until fork-tender.

Meanwhile, to make the lentil stew, heat the olive oil in a large, deep pot over medium heat. Add the carrots, onion, and celery and sauté until the vegetables are soft and the onionis translucent, about 5 minutes. Add the garlic and continue to cook for another 1 to 2 minutes, until fragrant. Add the paprika, cumin, turmeric, cinnamon, salt, and pepper and stir to combine.

Add the vegetable broth and stir, scraping the bottom of the pan to loosen all the browned bits. Add the lentils, stir, and cover the pan. Bring the mixture to a boil, then reduce the heat to medium-low and allow to simmer, covered, for 10 to 12 minutes, until the lentils are tender. Stir in the lemon juice and the kale and cook for 2 to 3 minutes, until wilted.

While the stew is simmering, finish the mashed potatoes. Drain and return them to the pot. Add the coconut cream, ghee, sea salt, and pepper. Mash the potatoes using a handheld mixer or potato masher if you like them chunky. Add the nondairy milk a few tablespoons at a time until you reach your desired consistency. Serve the mashed potatoes on a plate or bowl, ladle the stew over, and top with cilantro or parsley.

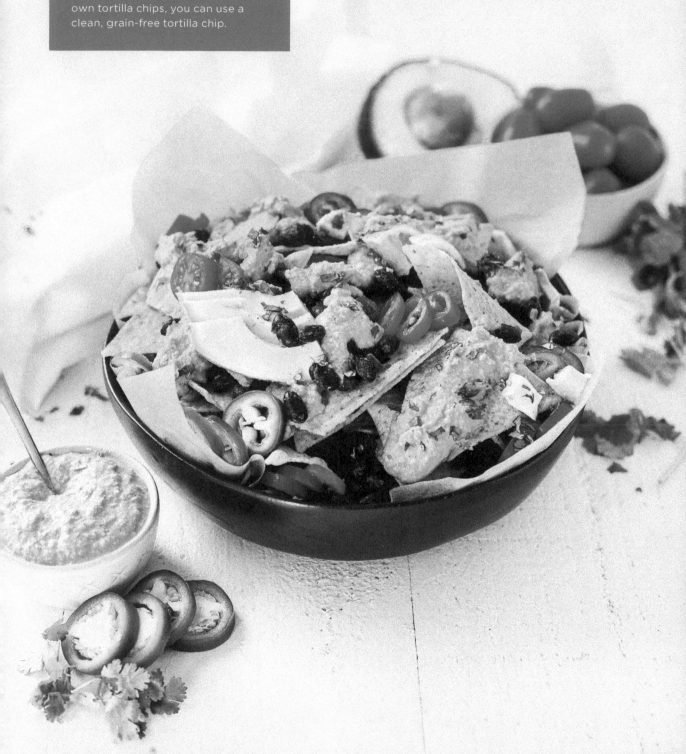

PRO TIP!

If you don't have time to make your own tortilla chips, you can use a clean, grain-free tortilla chip.

Spicy Black Bean Nachos with Cashew Queso

I can't resist nachos as an appetizer, but it's also fun to eat them as a main course. This recipe is just spicy enough, and loaded with fiber to keep you full.

For the nachos:

2 tablespoons (28 g) coconut oil

1 medium yellow onion, diced

2 garlic cloves, minced

1 (15-ounce/432 g) can black beans, rinsed and drained

1 (4-ounce/113 g) can diced green chiles, drained

1 teaspoon ground cumin

1 teaspoon smoked paprika

¼ teaspoon salt

¼ teaspoon cayenne pepper

6 ounces (170 g) clean corn or cassava tortilla chips

1 cup (180 g) cherry tomatoes, quartered

½ small red onion, diced

¼ cup (8 g) freshly chopped cilantro

1 small fresh jalapeño, sliced

1 medium avocado, peeled, pitted, and diced

For the cashew queso:

¾ cup (177 ml) hot water, plus more as needed

1 cup (145 g) raw cashews

⅓ cup (33 g) nutritional yeast

¼ cup (65 g) chunky salsa

1 garlic clove, peeled

½ teaspoon chili powder

½ teaspoon paprika

½ teaspoon ground cumin

½ teaspoon salt

—

Yield | 6 servings

Preheat the oven to 350°F (180°C). Line a rimmed baking sheet with parchment paper or aluminum foil.

To make the nachos, melt the coconut oil in a large, deep skillet over medium heat. Add the onion and cook, stirring frequently, for 2 to 3 minutes, until soft and translucent. Add the garlic and cook for another 1 to 2 minutes, until fragrant. Add the black beans, green chiles, cumin, smoked paprika, salt, and cayenne and cook, stirring frequently, for 2 to 3 more minutes.

Put half of the tortilla chips on the prepared baking sheet, top with half of the black bean mixture, then the remaining chips, and finally the remaining black beans. Bake for 10 minutes, or until the chips are heated through.

To make the cashew queso, combine all the cashew queso ingredients in a high-speed blender or food processor and blend on high until smooth and creamy, scraping down the sides as needed. If the queso is too thick, add more water, 1 tablespoon (15 ml) at a time.

Pour the queso over the chips and beans. Top with the cherry tomatoes, red onion, cilantro, jalapeños, and avocado. Serve immediately.

Mexican Street Corn Salad

Mexican night is our favorite, and this crunchy salad is a welcome change from traditional salads. It's spicy, sweet, and smoky—and there isn't any lettuce involved! The corn, bell pepper, onion, tomatoes, and fresh herbs make this a healthy and gluten-free side dish.

For the salad:

4 ears corn, shucked

1 tablespoon (15 ml) olive oil

1 teaspoon ground cumin

1 teaspoon chili powder

1 teaspoon salt

½ teaspoon black pepper

1 red bell pepper, seeded and diced

1 cup (180 g) cherry tomatoes, quartered

½ large onion, diced small

½ cup (16 g) minced fresh cilantro, plus more for garnish

For the dressing:

⅓ cup (75 g) paleo mayonnaise

¼ cup (58 ml) well-shaken canned full-fat coconut milk

2 tablespoons (32 g) mild salsa verde

2 teaspoons raw honey

2 teaspoons lime juice

¼ cup (34 g) pickled jalapeños

¼ cup (16 g) tightly packed fresh cilantro leaves and tender stems

1 garlic clove, peeled, or 1 teaspoon garlic powder

2 teaspoons dried chives

½ teaspoon salt

¼ teaspoon dried dill

⅛ teaspoon smoked paprika

—

Yield | 8 servings

Preheat the oven to 425°F (220°C).

To make the salad, rub each ear of corn with the olive oil and sprinkle with the cumin, chili powder, salt, and pepper. Wrap each ear individually in aluminum foil and place on a rimmed baking sheet. Bake for 20 minutes, turning halfway through.

To make the dressing, combine all the dressing ingredients in a food processor and blend on high for 1 to 2 minutes, until smooth and creamy. Set aside or refrigerate until ready to serve.

Combine the bell pepper, tomatoes, onion, and cilantro in a serving bowl. When the corn is done, unwrap the ears and allow them to cool. Stand each ear on its end in a shallow dish and cut the kernels off the cob. Add the corn to the salad and pour the dressing over the top. Mix well to coat everything. Garnish with additional cilantro.

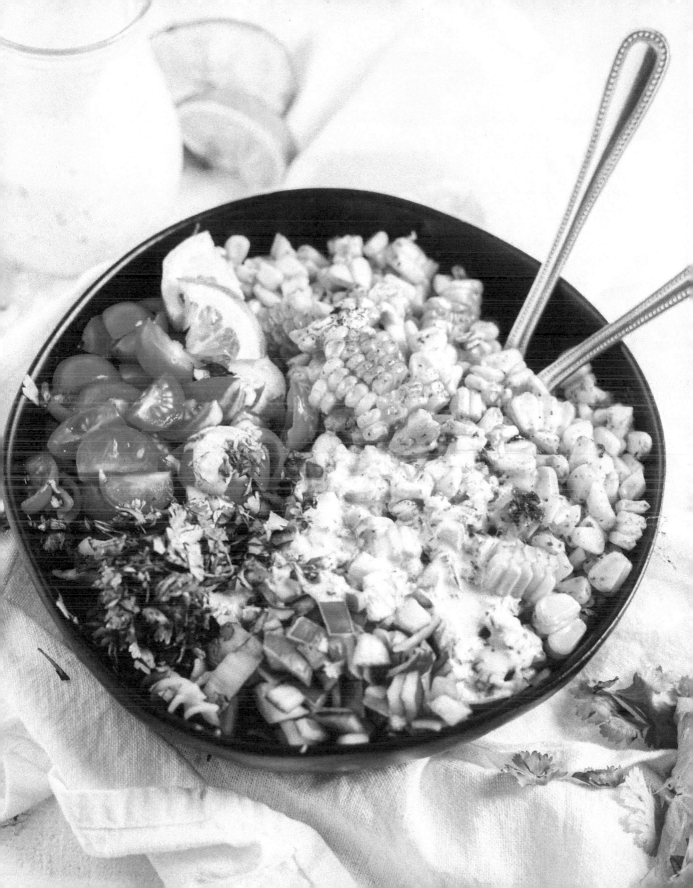

GF DF SF P V

Strawberry-Spinach Salad

This strawberry-spinach salad with poppy seed dressing is always a crowd-pleaser! It's made with homemade candied pecans, red onion, and a healthy dressing that takes just 5 minutes to make. Serve it as a side at dinnertime or add some cooked chicken for a healthy lunch.

For the candied pecans:

1 large egg white

¼ cup (85 g) pure maple syrup

1 teaspoon pure vanilla extract

1 teaspoon ground cinnamon

½ teaspoon salt

3 cups (300 g) pecans

For the salad:

10 cups (300 g) baby spinach

3 cups (510 g) sliced strawberries

½ small red onion, sliced

For the poppy seed dressing:

½ cup (118 ml) light olive oil or avocado oil

¼ cup (59 ml) white wine vinegar or champagne vinegar

¼ cup (85 g) raw honey

1 tablespoon (8 g) poppy seeds

2 teaspoons paleo mayonnaise

½ teaspoon ground mustard

½ teaspoon salt

—
Yield | 6 servings

Preheat the oven to 300°F (150°C). Line a rimmed baking sheet with parchment paper.

To make the candied pecans, in a medium bowl, whisk the egg white for 1 to 2 minutes, until frothy. Add the maple syrup, vanilla, cinnamon, and salt and gently stir. Add the pecans and fold them in until fully coated.

Pour out the pecans onto the prepared baking sheet. Spread into a single layer and bake for 20 to 25 minutes, stirring halfway through for even baking. You'll know they're done when the coating firms up and coats the pecans. Remove from the oven and allow to cool on the baking sheet until the pecans harden, about 15 minutes.

To make the salad, when the pecans have cooled, put the spinach in a large bowl and top with the strawberries, red onion, and pecans.

To make the dressing, combine all the dressing ingredients in a jar with a lid and shake well (or whisk together in a small bowl). Pour over the salad.

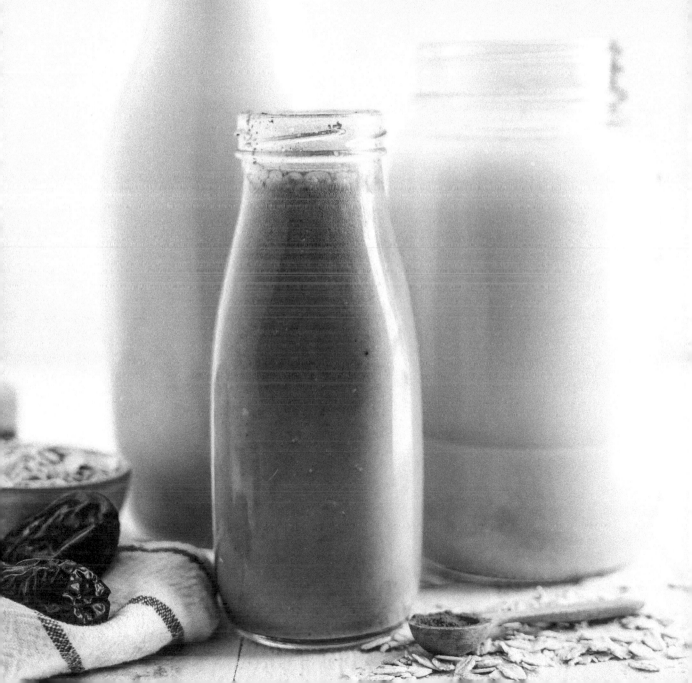

5-Minute Oat Milk, page 131

CHAPTER NINE

Beverages

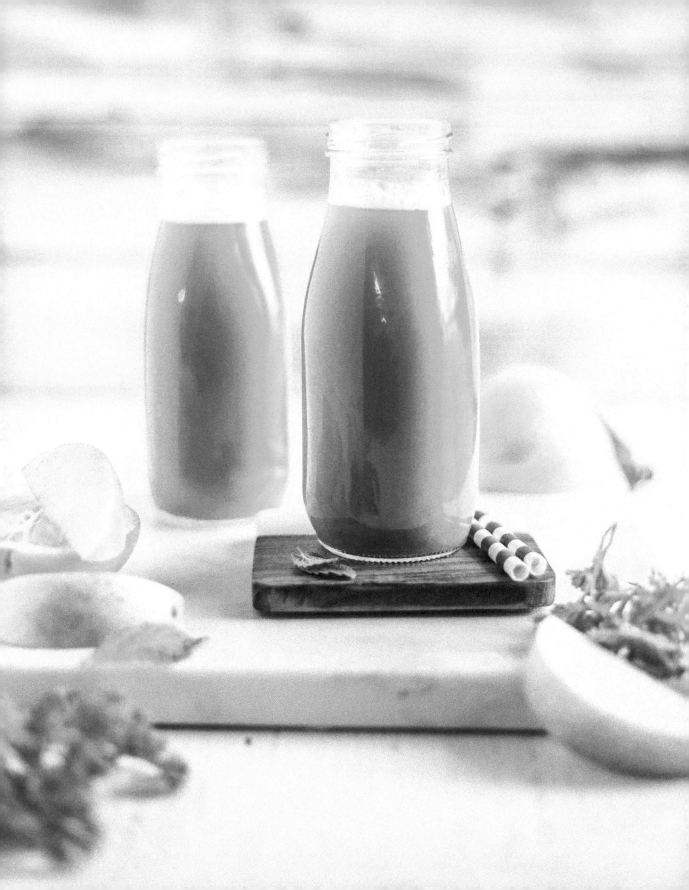

Kale Power Juice

Do you struggle to get all your greens throughout the day? I know it can be tough to fit them in, so I created this super simple green juice recipe—and it doesn't require a fancy juicer. All you need is a blender and nut milk bag or cheesecloth to make a batch to last you several days. It's a little sweet from the apple and pineapple, and the freshest (and healthiest!) thing you'll drink all day! If possible, try to use organic vegetables, and be sure to wash them well.

1½ cups (355 ml) water

Juice of 1 lemon

2 cups (134) chopped kale or 3 cups (90 g) baby spinach

1 cup (165 g) fresh or no-sugar-added canned pineapple chunks

2 celery stalks, roughly chopped

1 green apple, cored and cut into chunks

1 medium cucumber, cut into chunks

½ cup (30 g) fresh parsley leaves and tender stems

1 tablespoon (4 g) chopped fresh mint

1 (1-inch/2.5 cm) piece ginger, peeled and roughly chopped

—
Yield | 2 servings

Combine all the ingredients in a high-speed blender and blend on the highest setting for at least 1 minute, until completely combined.

Place a nut milk bag, thin kitchen towel, or cheesecloth over a large glass measuring cup or bowl. Pour the juice mixture into the bag, squeezing all the liquid into the bowl. Discard the pulp.

Drink immediately or store in an airtight container in the refrigerator for up to 2 days. Shake well before serving.

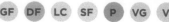

Cucumber-Mint-Celery Refresher

Fresh celery provides a multitude of vitamins, like K, C, and B[6] and celery juice has a high percentage of electrolytes to hydrate you, so that ingredient alone makes this bright and light drink a superfood. Add some ginger, lemon, and apple cider vinegar and you can't go wrong with drinking a glass of this every day. You'll feel like you can take on anything!

3 cups (710 ml) water

Juice of 1 lemon

3 tablespoons (45 ml) apple cider vinegar

4 celery stalks, roughly chopped

1 medium cucumber, cut into chunks

¼ cup (15 g) chopped fresh mint leaves and tender stems

¼ cup (15 g) chopped fresh parsley leaves and tender stems

1 (½-inch/1.25 cm) piece fresh ginger, peeled and roughly chopped

—
Yield | 4 cups (1185 ml)

Combine all the ingredients in a high-speed blender and blend on high for 3 to 4 minutes, until completely combined.

Place a nut milk bag, thin kitchen towel, or cheesecloth over a large glass measuring cup or bowl. Pour the juice mixture into the bag, squeezing all the liquid into the bowl. Discard the pulp.

Refrigerate for at least 30 minutes and serve cold.

PRO TIP!

If your ingredients are cold, you can add a cup of ice to the blender to chill the drink right away. Or serve over ice if you prefer!

5-Minute Oat Milk

Here's a nondairy milk alternative for all my nut-free friends! If you have a big bag of gluten-free rolled oats, you can whip up an affordable, creamy milk to add to granola, smoothies, coffee, and more.

2 cups (160 g) gluten-free rolled oats

2 quarts (1892 ml) water

1 teaspoon pure vanilla extract

1 teaspoon ground cinnamon

½ teaspoon salt

3 pitted Medjool dates or 3 tablespoons (60 g) pure maple syrup (optional)

—
Yield | 2 quarts (2 L)

ADD IT!

To make chocolate oat milk, add ¼ cup (30 g) raw cacao powder.

Combine all the ingredients in a high-speed blender and blend on high for 45 to 60 seconds, being careful not to overblend or the oats could become gummy.

Place a nut milk bag, thin kitchen towel, or cheesecloth over a large glass measuring cup or bowl. Pour the oat milk mixture into the bag, squeezing all the liquid into the bowl. Discard the oat pulp. If desired, strain the liquid a second time.

Use immediately or store in an airtight container in the refrigerator for up to 5 days. Shake well before serving.

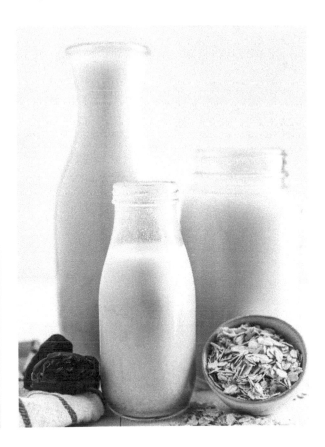

Mint Chocolate Chip Smoothie with Avocado

If you love mint chocolate chip ice cream, you'll love this creamy smoothie. The avocado adds a silky texture and healthy fats to keep you full. Use homemade oat milk for a smoothie that's completely made of whole foods and inflammation-fighting ingredients.

2 pitted Medjool dates

¾ cup (177 ml) 5-Minute Oat Milk (page 131) or other unsweetened nondairy milk, plus more as needed

½ medium avocado, peeled and pitted

1 cup (30 g) packed baby spinach

½ cup (66 g) frozen cauliflower florets

2 tablespoons (22 g) cocoa nibs

1 tablespoon (4 g) chopped fresh mint or ¼ teaspoon peppermint extract

¼ cup (65 g) ice

—

Yield | 1 smoothie

Put the dates in a small bowl, cover with hot water, and let soak for 5 minutes to soften. Drain, then transfer to a high-speed blender and add the remaining ingredients. Blend on high until smooth and creamy, scraping down the sides of the blender as needed. If you want it thinner, add up to ¼ cup (59 ml) more milk. Enjoy right away.

PRO TIP!

The frozen cauliflower chills this recipe and helps thicken it. If you don't have frozen cauliflower, add another ¼ cup (65 g) ice.

Strawberry-Cashew Smoothie

Cashews are full of polyunsaturated and monounsaturated fats, vitamin E, and minerals. They keep you full and add a mild flavor that goes well with the sweet strawberries and cauliflower. You're going to think you're drinking a strawberry milkshake!

1 pitted Medjool date

¾ cup (177 ml) cashew milk or other nondairy milk

1 cup (255 g) frozen strawberries

½ cup (66 g) frozen cauliflower florets

2 tablespoons (30 g) cashew butter

—

Yield | 1 smoothie

Put the date in a small bowl, cover with hot water, and let soak for 5 minutes to soften. Drain, then transfer to a high-speed blender and add the remaining ingredients. Blend on high for 2 to 3 minutes, until smooth and creamy. Enjoy right away.

PRO TIP!

You can use fresh strawberries if they're in season; just add ½ cup (130 g) ice to chill it and create a thick consistency.

 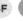
Agave Ginger Lemonade

Here we spice up traditional lemonade with a kick of fresh ginger. The agave is a refined sugar–free option to balance out the sour from the lemon. Gingerol, the main compound in fresh ginger, has powerful antioxidant and anti-inflammatory effects. You aren't just drinking lemonade on a hot day, you're fighting inflammation while you do it!

7 cups (1656 ml) water

¾ cup (255 g) agave or raw honey

1½ tablespoons (12 g) peeled and grated fresh ginger (a 4-inch/10 cm piece)

1 cup (237 ml) lemon juice (4 to 5 lemons)

Ice cubes, for serving

Yield | 4 servings

Combine the water, agave, and ginger in a medium saucepan and cook over medium-high heat, stirring frequently to dissolve the agave. Remove from the heat and strain out the ginger. Allow the liquid to come to room temperature. Add the lemon juice and serve over ice.

PRO TIP!

You can reduce the amount of agave depending on how sweet you like your lemonade.

Watermelon-Mint Mocktail

Citrus is rich in vitamin C, so the added orange and lime juice in this mocktail helps you fight inflammation on the hottest summer days. The texture is like a smooth slushy, and there's just a hint of mint flavor from the herb being infused in the simple syrup. I highly recommend keeping frozen watermelon on hand for anytime the craving strikes.

For the mint simple syrup:

½ cup (118 ml) water

¼ cup (85 g) raw honey or agave

¼ cup (16 g) roughly chopped fresh mint

For the mocktail:

6 cups (900 g) frozen watermelon

¼ cup (71 g) fresh squeezed orange juice (about 1 large navel orange)

2 tablespoons (30 ml) lime juice

1½ cups (390 g) ice

—
Yield | 4 servings

To make the mint simple syrup, heat the water and honey in a small saucepan over medium-high heat until the honey dissolves, about 3 minutes. Remove from the heat, add the chopped mint, cover, and set aside until the mixture comes to room temperature. Strain out the mint and discard.

To make the mocktail, transfer the mint simple syrup to a high-speed blender and add the mocktail ingredients. Blend on high until broken down and no large chunks of ice or watermelon remain. Serve immediately.

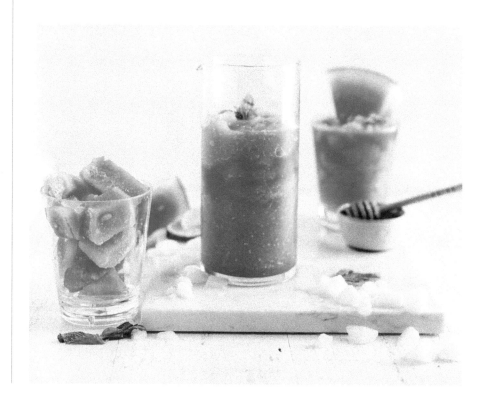

Very Berry Ginger Smoothie

You might not be able to pack any more anti-inflammatory ingredients into one recipe than this one! The ginger, berries, spinach, and cauliflower make this superfood smoothie a great way to start your day.

2 cups (60 g) spinach

2½ cups (591 ml) unsweetened nondairy milk, plus more as needed

1 frozen banana

2 cups (500 g) frozen mixed berries

½ cup (66 g) frozen cauliflower florets

2 tablespoons (30 g) almond butter

1 (1-inch/2.5 cm) piece fresh ginger, peeled

½ teaspoon ground cinnamon

—

Yield | 2 servings

Blend the spinach and milk in a high-speed on high for about 30 seconds. Add the remaining ingredients and blend for 1 minute, or until the smoothie is thick and creamy. Add more milk, 1 tablespoon (15 ml) at a time, if you want a thinner consistency. Enjoy right away.

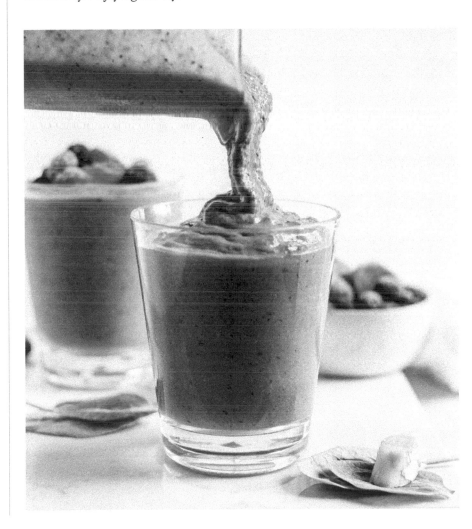

Vanilla Chai Latte

Ginger, cinnamon, and black pepper spice up this tea to give you the boost you need by mid-afternoon—all while fighting inflammation. There's so much flavor brimming in one spicy cup.

4 cups (946 ml) unsweetened nondairy milk

1 vanilla bean

3 tablespoons (60 g) pure maple syrup

4 black tea bags

1 teaspoon ground cinnamon, plus more for serving (optional)

½ teaspoon ground ginger

½ teaspoon ground nutmeg

½ teaspoon ground allspice

¼ teaspoon ground cardamom

¼ teaspoon ground cloves

⅛ teaspoon black pepper

Vanilla Bean Coffee Creamer (page 137), for serving (optional)

—
Yield | 2 servings

Pour the milk into a medium saucepan and heat over high heat. Slice the vanilla bean lengthwise and use the knife to scrape the vanilla seeds into the milk. Stir to combine. Heat the milk until scalding, but not boiling, about 5 minutes. Remove the pan from the heat, add the maple syrup and tea bags, and steep for 5 minutes.

Add the cinnamon, ginger, nutmeg, allspice, cardamom, cloves, and pepper and whisk to combine or use a hand frother to mix and froth the milk. Serve hot with coffee creamer, and an extra sprinkling of cinnamon, if you like.

ADD IT!

If you can't find vanilla beans, use 1 teaspoon pure vanilla extract. Add it at the same time as the maple syrup.

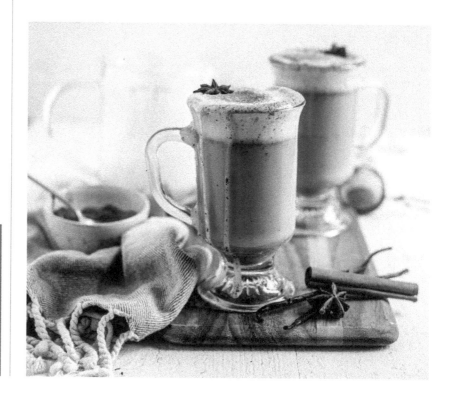

Creamy Hot Cocoa

Cold nights call for cozy cups of rich and creamy hot cocoa. Get creative for the season with almond extract, peppermint extract, or a dusting of pumpkin pie spice.

1 (13.5-ounce/383 g) can full-fat coconut milk

⅓ cup (79 ml) unsweetened nondairy milk

½ cup (88 g) dairy-free chocolate chips

1 tablespoon (8 g) unsweetened cocoa powder

½ teaspoon pure vanilla extract

⅛ teaspoon salt

—
Yield | 2 servings

In a medium saucepan over medium heat, whisk together the coconut milk and nondairy milk for about 1 minute. Add the chocolate chips, cocoa powder, vanilla, and salt and whisk until the chocolate is melted and smooth. Mix and stir until the mixture is heated through but not boiling. Serve immediately.

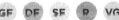

GF DF SF P VG V

Vanilla Bean Coffee Creamer

If you love a good cup of dairy-free creamy coffee in the morning, make your own! This simple cashew creamer features raw nuts, a real vanilla bean, and creamy coconut milk. Make a batch each weekend for coffee creamer all week.

8 ounces (227 g) raw cashews

2 pitted Medjool dates

2½ cups (591 ml) water

½ vanilla bean

½ cup (115 ml) canned full-fat coconut milk, shaken well before measuring

⅛ teaspoon salt

—
Yield | 3½ cups (830 ml)

Put the cashews and dates in a medium bowl and cover with hot water. Allow to soak for 1 hour at room temperature. Drain and transfer the cashews and dates to a high-speed blender. Add the water and blend on high for 3 to 4 minutes, until the cashews are broken up and you can no longer see any chunks.

Place a nut milk bag, thin kitchen towel, or cheesecloth over a large glass measuring cup or bowl. Pour the cashew milk mixture into the bag, squeezing all the liquid into the bowl. Discard the cashew pulp. If desired, strain the liquid a second time.

Pour the milk back into the blender. Slice the vanilla bean lengthwise and use the knife to scrape the vanilla seeds into the blender. Add the coconut milk and salt and blend for 30 seconds, or until smooth. Store in an airtight jar in the refrigerator.

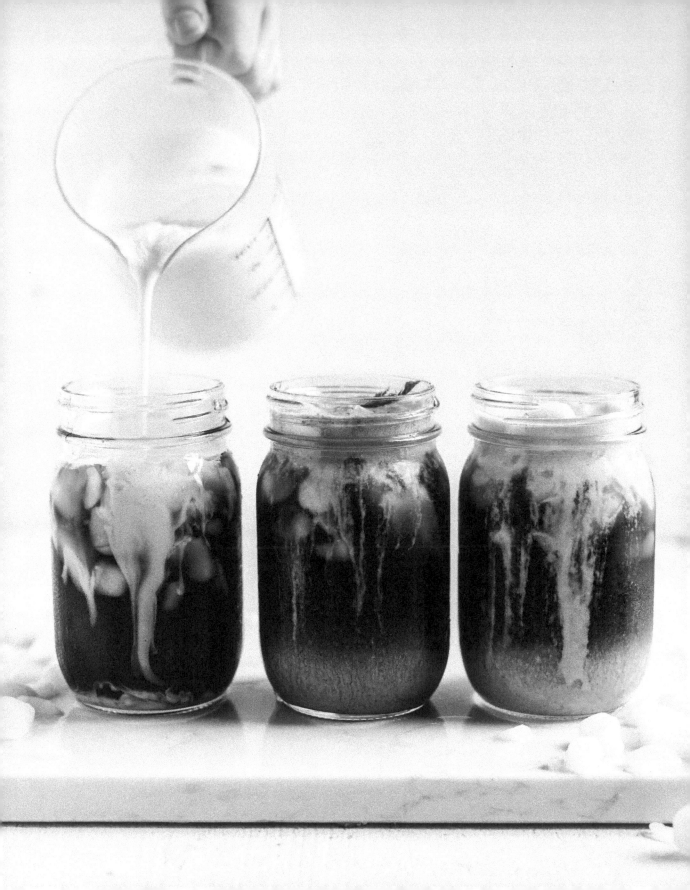

Bulletproof Iced Coffee 3 Ways

Bulletproof coffee is a blend of brewed coffee and healthy fats. This recipe is made with MCT oil to boost energy and support cognitive function as well as coconut milk to keep you full and satisfied in the morning. The addition of collagen helps improve gut health, balances blood sugar, and supports healthy skin and nails. Customize this simple recipe with whatever you're craving, and your delicious morning coffee turns into a superfood start to your day.

For the cream base:

1 (13.5-ounce/383 g) can full-fat coconut milk

½ cup (118 ml) unsweetened nondairy milk

3 tablespoons (60 g) pure maple syrup

2 tablespoons (30 ml) MCT oil

1 teaspoon pure vanilla extract

2 tablespoons (10 g) collagen powder

½ teaspoon salt

For the mint mocha variation:

1 teaspoon unsweetened cocoa powder

½ teaspoon peppermint extract

Fresh mint leaves, for garnish

For the pumpkin spice variation:

1 tablespoon (15 g) canned pumpkin puree

½ teaspoon pumpkin pie spice

For the spiced Thai variation:

¼ teaspoon almond extract

¼ teaspoon ground cardamom

Ice cubes, for serving

2½ cups (591 ml) cold-brewed coffee

—

Yield | 2 servings

To make the cream base, combine all the cream base ingredients in a high-speed blender. Add the ingredients for whichever flavor variation you're choosing and blend on high for 30 to 60 seconds, until smooth and creamy.

Fill 2 large glasses with ice and divide the cold-brew coffee evenly between them. Pour the flavored cream over the coffee and stir. Enjoy right away!

Golden Turmeric-Honey Latte

Manuka honey is a type of honey native to New Zealand, produced by bees that pollinate the manuka bush. It's most widely known for its antibacterial properties, and specifically for improving gut health—a critical piece to healing chronic inflammation as a whole. If you can, use this honey for extra anti-inflammatory benefits in this soothing recipe. However, the turmeric, ginger, cinnamon, and pepper alone make this a powerful healing combination.

2 cups (473 ml) unsweetened nondairy milk

1 tablespoon (20 g) manuka honey

1 teaspoon grated and peeled fresh ginger

2½ teaspoons ground turmeric

1 teaspoon ground cinnamon, plus more for topping (optional)

⅛ teaspoon black pepper

—
Yield | 2 servings

Combine all the ingredients in a blender and blend on high until combined. Place a nut milk bag, thin kitchen towel, or cheesecloth over a small saucepan and strain the mixture to remove any bits of ginger. Heat the mixture over high heat until scalding, about 5 minutes. Enjoy with an additional sprinkle of cinnamon, if you like.

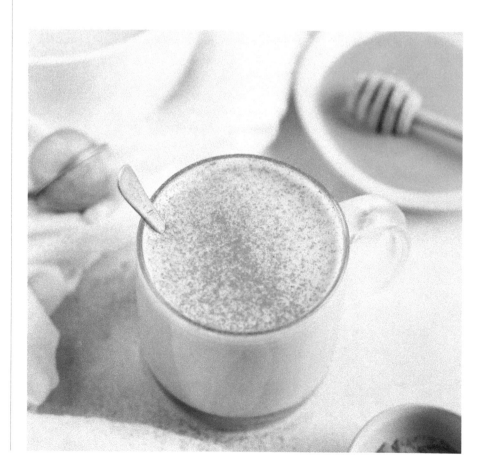

Acknowledgments

To my What Molly Made community, you're the reason I do what I do. Thank you for allowing me to be a small part of your journey. You've liked, saved, tried, and shared my recipes and have allowed me to turn my passion into a career.

Zach, you changed my life for the better. This book wouldn't be possible without you. You are my rock and this book is as much yours as it is mine. Thanks for being my permanent taste tester and my very best friend.

Cooper, you've given me a purpose I didn't know existed. My hope is that I can teach you to have a healthy relationship with food—one that nourishes your body, gathers our family, and helps celebrate the best moments in life. Thanks for being a good sleeper so Mom could rest up for recipe testing!

Mom and Dad, your love and support mean so much. I was so scared about making What Molly Made my full-time job, but you told me to take the leap, then bought me a new camera. I believe in myself because you believe in me. You don't get to choose your family, but I'd choose you over and over.

Kaleigh and Elisa, you're my big sisters and I look up to you so much. Thanks for putting up with all the recipe pictures I send. Your love and friendship have impacted me in ways that go beyond sisterhood.

Nana, DaddyBob, and Nama, thank you for creating a family that loves, forgives, celebrates, and supports each other. You're the foundation of our family and I love you.

To the Thompsons and Niemans, I got lucky and gained another loving and supportive family. The way you all gather around the table for quality time is something that will stick with me forever.

To our One Church family, this cookbook-writing season wouldn't have happened without the way you showed up for us. The texts, calls, babysitting, and hugs touched our hearts and made all the recipes in this book possible.

Chelsea and Cathy Shew, thanks for buying me my first cookbook and teaching me how to make things like beef tenderloin and bananas Foster.

Amanda and Lydia, I'm grateful for your support and guidance as my editors. You helped me manifest this book from ideas in my head to printed pages in reader's hands.

Julie Gratmeyer, you helped me heal from the inside out and helped me finally feel understood. Thanks for guiding me through this anti-inflammatory journey.

About the Author

Molly Thompson is the founder of the popular website What Molly Made (whatmollymade.com), where she focuses on easy, healthy recipes that use natural ingredients, often fitting into special diets like gluten free, paleo, or anti-inflammatory. Molly also shares her own personal story about living with PCOS on her blog, and how she uses an anti-inflammatory diet to reverse symptoms naturally. Her site also specializes in recipe development, professional food photography, and video production.

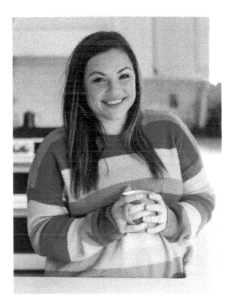

Index

CPSIA information can be obtained
at www.ICGtesting.com
Printed in the USA
BVHW061253190123
656172BV00008B/9